How to do Everything and be Happy

Your step-by-step, straight-talking guide to creating happiness in your life

Peter Jones

HarperCollins*Publishers*

HarperCollins*Publishers*
77–85 Fulham Palace Road,
Hammersmith, London W6 8JB

www.harpercollins.co.uk
www.howtodoeverythingandbehappy.com

First published in the UK by soundhaven.com 2011
This edition published by HarperCollins*Publishers* 2013

13 5 7 9 10 8 6 4 2

Text © Peter Jones 2011

Peter Jones asserts the moral right to be
identified as the author of this work

A catalogue record of this book is
available from the British Library

ISBN 978-0-00-750194-6

FSC™ is a non-profit international organisation established to promote
the responsible management of the world's forests. Products carrying the
FSC label are independently certified to assure consumers that they come
from forests that are managed to meet the social, economic and
ecological needs of present and future generations,
and other controlled sources.

Find out more about HarperCollins and the environment at
www.harpercollins.co.uk/green

In memory of Kate,
her Big Theory of Everything,
and all the amazing things she taught me.
Love, as always,
Peter

Contents

To Begin With …

Once upon a time I got sold a dream: I would grow up big and strong, marry a blonde (my mother was convinced of this), have children, and live happily ever after in a big house, whilst I held down a job as an astronaut. Or a train driver. Or a fireman. And this wasn't a 'maybe' – something to aspire to – this was my God-given right. This is what was going to happen. All I had to do was wait.

Not that I was very good at waiting. I'm still not very good at waiting! I wanted this idyllic life now. I didn't want to wait until *next week* or some other distant point in the future.

I must have told my parents this because they would smile and tell me not to be in such a rush. 'Peter,' they would say, 'schooldays are the best days of your life.'

Obviously they were mistaken. They had to be. When my parents' eyes glazed over and they talked fondly of 'schooldays', they must have been recalling the days of their own distant childhood, days sitting around camp fires outside the school mud hut, marking bits of slate with chalk whilst village elders told stories of dragons. Their schooldays were clearly a far cry from the mixture of humiliation, bullying and boredom that I endured. They had to be. Because if they weren't, for schooldays to be the 'best' days they would logically have to be followed by 'something worse'.

Then I got older, and things got worse.

Actually, that's not quite true. They didn't get any worse – not really – but they certainly didn't get much better, and they definitely got more complex.

'Work' turned out to be very similar to 'school' –
different bullies, same rules, just as boring. And whereas I
was given money in return for surrendering five days out of
seven – more money than I'd ever dreamed possible –
now there was a slew of people lining up to take it away
from me.

And then there were relationships. Just when I'd got
classroom note passing down to a fine art, the game changed
completely, and note passing wasn't going to cut it.

I could go on, but suffice it to say, the initial 'dream'
seemed less and less likely. It was clear that I was never going
to be an astronaut. Or a train driver. Or a fireman. It also
seemed unlikely that I would ever live in a big house. Big
houses needed big money. I was on small to medium money.
Two bedroom flat money.

Finally, on my thirty-second birthday, I realised there was
a distinct possibility that I might never ever find 'the blonde'.

This was a serious blow. Without the blonde I might
never be married, I might never have children – and whilst I
could probably cope without being married or having kids,
or my blonde actually being a blonde, I couldn't imagine
being single for the rest of my days. That was unacceptable.
Something had to be done.

So, for the first time in my life, I started to plan – to
make lists, and take control of my own destiny. Many of the
techniques in this book are nothing more than the skills I had
to develop to avoid a life of bachelorhood. But it worked.
Eventually I found the blonde. Took me a few more years,
considerable effort on my part, and a somewhat unorthodox
approach to dating, but I found her.

And we did marry.

And when she died in my arms three years later I was heartbroken.

People rarely ask me how Kate died. It's just not the sort of question they feel comfortable asking. Most assume she must have had cancer – that we'd have had some warning. We didn't.

I was off to our place in Croatia for a few days to finish my novel. Kate drove me to the airport and as she dropped me off she gave me the world's biggest hug, bit back a few tears, thumped me in the arm, and told me she loved me – and that I'd better call her when I got to the other end.

I walked towards the main airport building, turned to give her one last wave. Something wasn't right.

I could see our car, but not her.

The next few hours are a bit of a blur. I remember dropping my bags and running back to our vehicle. Taking her in my arms. The lady police officer trying to revive her. I remember the paramedics, the ambulance helicopter, being rushed to the hospital in the back of a police car. And I remember that god-awful waiting room, the stony faces of the doctors as they told me there was nothing they could do, that my wife was gone, and that they'd be switching off the life support machine.

Several hours later I drove our car back to an empty house.

I've learned since that deaths like this (a sub-arachnoid haemorrhage, according to the certificate) are surprisingly common. Kate had had a weak part in her brain, probably since birth, and it could have happened at any moment. It was almost inevitable.

I've learned too that after the shock comes the guilt. Every cross word, every nasty thought, every lie – they all come back to haunt you. And amongst the demons that were lining up to torment me was the realisation that I wasn't happy, and maybe I never had been.

There had been happy moments, of course. Quite a lot of moments. Most of them in the previous three years, and most of them down to Kate, but they were moments nonetheless. I wanted to be happy all the time. Not just occasionally. Not just for a moment. And for the second time in my life I decided to tackle a problem in the only way I knew how: by making plans, and lists, and taking control of my own destiny.

Welcome to *How to Do Everything and Be Happy!*

If you're dissatisfied with your life, this book may be for you.

If you want to do something – anything – to increase the amount of happiness you feel, this book is probably for you.

And if you know how to use a pencil, if you own a diary, if you can make a list, if you're moderately organised, or could be if you had a good enough reason to be, then this book is definitely for you.

Now then, let me tell you about this dream that I have for you …

Why the Long Face?

General Unhappiness

It's 9am on a Monday morning. The sky is a threatening mix of greys. The wind has slammed every door in the house, taken the lid off the bin, thrown it down the street, and is now attempting to wrestle the trees to the ground. Meanwhile the rain is pounding against the window like it's trying to get in. It's not what you need right now, and none of it is doing anything to soothe your hangover. Or is it a headache? Either way, your head pounds as if your skull is slowly being crushed in a vice, and all you can do to ease the pain is rub your eyes – eyes that feel like someone rolled them in chalk dust whilst you slept. All you have to do is make it till lunchtime, and then – maybe – you can sneak out to the car and get your head down for 15 minutes.

Except that it's not Monday morning. It's Wednesday afternoon. On a balmy spring day. The sky's finally realised that when it comes to clouds, less is most definitely more. The only wind is a gentle breeze that carries the sounds of the children from the school opposite. It's only Monday morning inside your head.

But that's how you feel all the time. Or most of the time. Enough that it bugs you. Enough that you picked up a book on happiness.

And it's how I used to feel.

Right now, as I write this book, I estimate 92% of my life was spent being 'unhappy'.[1] Not in an 'active' way, just – you know – a bit fed up with life. I had my share of moments where I stared at the cards life had dealt me and wondered how it was possible that there wasn't a single ace or picture card in my hand. I was 'a bit disappointed with it all'. There was a general lack of happiness in my days. I was un-happy.

In other words, I was, and very occasionally still am, pretty much like you, and most of the people we know. One of my closest friends once described it like this: 'I'm not,' he said, 'living the life I would have chosen for myself.'

So what's the cause?

Obviously there are numerous reasons. Therapists, psychologists and sociologists can probably carve them up and categorise them in numerous ways, but there are just three that seem right to me.

Let's take a closer look at General Unhappiness.

---

1 My assistant asked me how on earth I came up with that figure. Then before I could answer she said, 'You created a spreadsheet, didn't you!' I'm ashamed to admit it, but yes – I did.

Cause Number 1: Lousy Work/Life Balance

According to 'popular wisdom', no one lies on their death bed and thinks to themselves, 'I really wish I'd spent more time at work.'

Or do they?

Perhaps, out there, there's some lucky fellow who has, or had, this amazing job, and they either did, or are likely to, lie on their death bed and wish they'd spent more time in the office. Who could that person be?

Let's consider some possible candidates:

CONTESTANT NUMBER 1:

TOM HANKS

A-LIST HOLLYWOOD ACTOR

You know, I bet even Mr Hanks gets fed up with being an A-list Hollywood Actor. It's not all glitz, you know. For one thing, there's the paparazzi, constantly hounding Britney Spears and ignoring Tom. What exactly does an A-list actor have to do to get his picture on the front of a few magazines these days? Where's the respect? What happened to the days when raw talent was enough to get you noticed? Nowadays those press guys are only interested in shoving a camera in your face when you're face down in a puddle of something foul.

Will Tom be wishing he spent more time at work when the time comes to visit the big awards ceremony in the sky? Not a chance.

CONTESTANT NUMBER 2:
BILL GATES
CREATOR OF MICROSOFT

Being the second richest man on the planet[2] must be quite a buzz.

Thing is though, even if Bill decided to phone in sick, and to lie in bed for the rest of his life, he'd still be amongst the richest people that have ever lived – he doesn't actually have to *work* at it any more.

Now he might lie on his death bed and have regrets about Windows 95, Windows Vista, and Office 2007 – as well he should – but that would be a desire to atone for his crimes to humanity. In many ways those heinous errors of judgement might have actually been avoided if Bill had stayed at home once in a while. So when the time comes and Dr Watson walks into the room to tell Bill that there's been an unexpected error in his Life and it needs to Shut Down, will he wish he'd spent more time at the office?

No.

Next.

CONTESTANT NUMBER 3:
JULIO CASI AMOREO
WORLD'S GREATEST LOVER,
MALE ESCORT &
FIGMENT OF PETER JONES'S IMAGINATION

---

2 At the time of writing.

Maybe there's someone out there who gets paid to make love to the world's most fabulously gorgeous women. (What? It could happen!)

On his death bed in his villa, somewhere in southern Italy, surrounded by beautiful, grief-stricken lovers, Julio looks around him and, as a gentle breeze wafts in through the window and plays with his hair, he realises that even though he was managing three or four ladies, every day, for the past twenty years, he still failed to get to them all.

Maybe Julio will wish he'd worked more.

Well done. We thought of someone. Though we had to make him up. And you and I are probably in the minority for believing such a job can be described as 'work'.

Actually, it occurs to me that we probably need to take a moment to define what 'work' is.

This isn't the dictionary definition, but it's one that feels right to me:

Work is:
- Anything you <u>have</u> to do (be that earning money, picking the kids up from school, paying bills, sorting through your post, chores, family commitments ...)
- Doing whatever it is you *need* to do to sustain your life (earning money, robbing banks, living off the land ...)

And, this being the case, here are some interesting things I've noticed about 'work':
- Most of us are conditioned to believe that we <u>must</u> work. (Sure, many of us *have* to work, to earn money

for food, clothes, and to keep a home running – but the conditioning is actually a belief that we <u>must</u> work, and that we're lazy, or stupid, or not pulling our weight if we don't.)

- Work tends to fill the space available.
- Some smart aleck decided that the average working week should be five days out of seven. Five out of seven!

This being the case it's ridiculously easy to end up with a situation where work totally dominates your life. Where it's virtually the only thing you do during waking hours.

Try this simple exercise:

Taking no more than thirty seconds, think of three things you did in the last twenty-four hours that don't fall under my definition of 'work'.

So, you're done? What were your three things?

Were they …

1. eating,
2. watching TV, and
3. sleeping?

If you had something better on your list (I'll let you off if you 'went out for dinner') did it take you more than thirty seconds to come up with your list?

Now, I'm not suggesting for one moment that work isn't necessary and is somehow a *bad* thing. I'm not proposing that we eliminate work. Work is necessary. But for most people the balance of work and 'everything else' in their life is all wrong. And in many cases the 'everything else' lacks substance.

Reader 'Anon' emailed me:

'I'm sure a lot of us are in a job we don't enjoy for one reason or another, and let's face it, the recession has left us well and truly stuck – it seems far too scary to leave the secure job we have, even if it does make us miserable! I was wondering if you had any practical tips on how to survive doing things which make us unhappy but that we HAVE TO do? Is there a way of finding happiness in a job when we can't stand our work colleagues or are treated badly by the powers above? Thanks Peter.'

'Dear Anon,

Not that long ago I used to work in the banking industry. I spent my days telling rich men how to get richer by making poor people poorer. I used to leave the house in the morning and make some passing quip to my wife about how I was off to torture some souls. She'd ask me if I'd forgotten my pitch fork and horns. Like so many things said in jest, it wasn't actually very funny.

Finally, two years ago I couldn't take it any more. I went back to see the therapist who helped me through the loss of my wife, and six months later I finally summoned the courage to leave the security of a regular pay cheque behind.

Financially it's been a tough few months. And as I write this now I'm not quite out of the woods. My outgoings still outweigh my income but ... I have a plan. If things keep going the way they have been I should be supporting myself as a full-time author by the end of the year.

So my dear Anon, whoever you may be, it can be done. You can change your life. I don't believe in rash decisions, or risking everything ... but life's too short not to try.

"Survival" shouldn't be your first option.

Best wishes,

Peter'

If, like Anon, 'work' has become something you feel you need to 'survive', there are three obvious ways to improve your work-life balance:

1. Work less
2. Improve the non-work portion of your life
3. Make work fun (which might involve changing the very nature of what 'work' is)

I've tried – and am still trying – all three approaches. Maybe you instinctively know that one or all of these might work for you, but try not to get fixated on that right now. Keep that thought in the back of your mind, or better still, *jot it on a piece of paper*. We'll come back to it later.

In the meantime let's move on to the second reason for General Unhappiness.

Cause Number 2: Lack of Control

Run down the following list and keep a count in your head of the number of times you say, 'Yes, that applies to me.'

1. Other people have a say in how your life works.
2. *Everyone* else gets a say in how your life works.
3. You feel powerless a lot of the time.
4. Everyone, and everything else, comes first.
5. You say things like 'I can't do {what I want}, because I've got to do ...'
6. What you want (to do) is right at the bottom of your to-do list.
7. Your to-do list is mainly a list of items given to you by someone else.
8. You say things like 'Things will be so much better when ...'
9. This isn't the life you would have chosen for yourself.
10. You find yourself jealously protecting the half-an-hour you have to yourself each day ...
11. ... or the one night a week when you go to your evening class, club, pub etc.
12. You have secret friends, hobbies, lovers, possessions ... anything, just something that you can call *yours*.

How did you score? I scored one, perhaps one and a half. A few years back I would have scored a nine, maybe even a ten.

Things were pretty miserable back then: I would get up really early in the morning just so I could be on my own. I would go to work an hour earlier than was strictly necessary, and I'd take the scenic route there. Once at work I'd count the hours till lunchtime, and then again till I could leave. Then I'd drive the long way home, a different route this time, with a certain amount of dread about what awaited me when I got in.

Once home I'd get cross if there was anything that needed my attention – something to fix, a phone call to make, or even post to open. I'd get cross if there was nothing for dinner. I'd get cross if I couldn't watch television (though I didn't care what was on). And I'd definitely get cross if I couldn't have a glass of wine. Particularly as I wanted two. And after all this crossness I'd go to bed. Ridiculously early.

My days would be spent impatiently waiting for the next 'bit', just so whatever I was currently doing would end.

I'd spend weekdays longing for the weekend, and the weekend longing for Monday morning.

And I spent hours and hours wishing. I made long secret lists of wishes: 'Things I would do someday …' Except someday never came. My only purpose in life was to make sure my body was where it was supposed to be at an allotted time. I was a prisoner inside my own existence.

And the really sad thing is, I wasn't the only one. My wife felt like that too. We were both slaves to a growing number of responsibilities that controlled our every waking hour.

So who was holding us to ransom? Who was pulling the strings? Who was the evil mastermind behind the wicked forces in our lives?

We were.

We let it happen. And it wasn't hard to do.

What's more, we thought it was a phase. A blip. Something to get through. Good times were just around the corner, and if they weren't, we still had the rest of our lives for things to get better.

And whilst that might be true for me, it wasn't for my wife.

If I could jump back in time and tell my younger self that I'd only be with Kate for three years and three months, and that those would be the very last moments she would have on this planet, I'd change everything. Right away.

In short: *I'd have made every damn day count.*

Let's get one thing straight here. You can't 'live every day as though it's your last'. That's impractical. Stupid, even. But you *can* grab back the reins of your life, get back in the driving seat, and take back control. It's not easy. There'll be resistance. Lots of it. The majority of it from yourself. But my God, you'll feel better.

'Terrific!' you might be thinking. 'Another self-help book that wants to tell me how the unhappiness I feel is my fault! What a load of baloney! Can I get a refund?'

Relax.

This book's being written by an Englishman, and as such it's finally time to start pointing the finger at others.

Cause Number 3: External Forces

Sometimes the thing that's making you unhappy is staring
you right in the face. People might tell you that you need to
relax, calm down, try not to take things personally, roll with
the punches, 'make lemonade when life gives you lemons',
but sometimes that's not going to cut it.
Sometimes, it isn't you.

Sometimes it really is *them*.

Let's take a look at who *they* are.

For me, 'Other People' have more power than anything else
to drain my enthusiasm and suck the pleasure out of life.

It isn't always the people you think it would be either.
Sure, the angry idiot who gestured at me from his car as he
drove past took the edge off what might have been a pleasant
drive home, but he's soon forgotten, and I can take solace in
the fact that by the way he's driving he'll probably wrap his
car around a tree in the not too distant future.

No, the people who really have the power to make me
unhappy are either people who I care about, or people who
are, in some way, important in my life.

We all have them: The manager you don't get on with
– one who seems intent on making your life a misery. The
ex-partner you still have to see at family gatherings. The
moody work colleague you have to tiptoe around. Or the aged
relative who you love dearly, but has started to take you for
granted.

Occasionally it isn't the interaction with these people
that drives us crazy, but the lack thereof. Like the client

or a supplier who never returns your calls, never answers your emails, and is somehow never in the office when you 'pop by'. Or the friend or sibling who is so wrapped up in themselves that after an hour or so in their company you really begin to wonder whether all you are is some sort of audience.

Then there are the corporations, companies and government bodies that determine the structure in which we live, and rarely does a day go by when I haven't got to deal with some browbeaten call centre representative from an organisation that actually doesn't give two figs about whatever my plight might be. You might be forgiven for wondering if these organisations are run by people whose entire aim in life is to make as much money as possible, by any means, but without bringing the *slightest* bit of joy to anyone involved in the process. Having worked for a number of such organisations I can divulge that this is indeed the case.

Shortly after writing the first edition of this book, I started running *How to Do Everything and Be Happy* workshops.[3] They're a lot of fun, and because they're mainly attended by Brits, one of the most popular elements of the course seems to be when I give the group the opportunity to suggest what would make their 'External Forces' list. Here's just a sample of some of the more popular culprits:

- My job (see General Unhappiness Reason Number 1)

- Call centres
- Idiot drivers
- Parking (or lack of)
- Taxes
- Mondays
- My ex
- My hormones
- Rubbish TV
- People who walk in front of me very, very slowly
- Lateness (mine or other people's)
- Not getting enough sleep
- Pre-recorded call centre messages – 'We're experiencing a high volume of calls at the moment' – no you're not! This is the same volume of calls you've had for the past ten years!
- The road works we've had outside my building for the past ten weeks!
- Unfairness
- Bags of lettuce (why isn't it possible to buy a bloody head of lettuce any more?!)
- 'If your call is about something trivial, press 1. If your call is related to something else trivial, press 2. If your call is related to a trivial matter not related to the first two trivial matters press 3. If your call …'
- Clients who yell at me when there's nothing I can do about it
- The UK winter (being dark at 4pm)
- Friends letting me down or losing touch with friends
- Family not 'understanding' me or saying something that makes me feel low

- 'Did you know you can check your balance on our website?' Yes, I did! Put me through to a real person!
- Having a fat day, or bad hair day
- Being broke (worrying about money)
- Stressing about 'my life'
- Family or friends being sick or ill, i.e. worrying about them
- Not having enough time with my family
- Not having a holiday
- Being stuck in the house
- Fines, e.g. bank fees, parking tickets, etc
- Having to go to the doctor
- Paying for a coffee then finding that it's rubbish (same goes for a sub-standard meal, or bad service)
- The news
- Thinking about climate change
- Littering
- Other people's children
- Walking past homeless people
- Boredom
- Mess, that I have to clean up
- Procrastination (makes me guilty, then consequently blue)

Doubtless you'll have your own items. The question is – what can you do about it? How can you reduce the power these things have over you?

Stop right there!

That way lies madness.

After Kate died one of the first things I did on my 'quest to find happiness' was to compile a list very similar to the one above, and then work through it, tackling each item head on with a view to eliminating my unhappiness. I even invented a misery rating so that I could re-sort it and go after the big hitters first.

I soon discovered two things:

Firstly, it didn't matter how hard I worked, I just never seemed to make a big enough dent in that damn list. I was forever adding new items! I felt like a guy in a leaky rowing boat – going nowhere fast whilst desperately trying to get rid of the water that won't stop coming in.

Secondly, pretty soon the list itself became something I hated. I ended up calling it my 'Ugh List', because that's how it made me feel: Ugh! Every moment I spent focusing on the list was more time involved with things that made me unhappy. (We'll be coming back to how the mind deals with focus later in the book, so keep that thought at the back of your mind.)

I'm pleased to report however that the Ugh List did teach me one, very valuable, lesson:

THE ABSENCE OF UNHAPPINESS
IS NOT HAPPINESS

The more I worked on the list the more I came to realise that even if I managed to eliminate all my Ugh items there was a very real chance that I still wouldn't be happy. Happiness, it seems, just doesn't work that way.

Whilst it might be mildly interesting to list the reasons for your unhappiness (and quite seductive too – there's a part of us that *wants* to do that), I've come to suspect that the *true* cause of unhappiness might actually be the absence of happiness.

Which is very good news.

Because it turns out, happiness isn't all that difficult to find.

Doing Something About It

Let's recap.

The top three reasons for General Unhappiness (according to me anyway) are:

Lousy Work/life Balance
Where the things you *have* to do dominate your life, and the things you'd *like* to do just aren't meaty enough, or you don't have enough of them, to 'balance' your life.

A General Lack of Control
Where you find yourself bouncing around the pinball machine of life, and you're not in control of the flippers.

External Forces
Where you encounter people or situations that seem intent on taking your sunny smiley mood and crushing it into the ground.

Now, would you like to do something about it?

During the pages that follow I'll take you through practical steps to (re)organise your life so that you increasingly find yourself doing things that make you happy, and spending less time churning through the stuff that sucks the joy out of life.

Putting the smile back on your face won't necessarily involve identifying problem areas of your life and attempting to 'fix' or eliminate them. But, that said, we are going to improve your work/life balance. We're also going to snatch back control of your life and put you back in the driving seat. And finally we will start redesigning your life so that those external influences either won't seem so influential, or won't be there at all.

This book's designed to get you started right away. Seven days is really all you need. That's the minimum time required to read the book, and to start putting some of the ideas into practice. We'll start with the easy stuff and build on it. If you work with me as we go through the various chapters you'll feel much happier by this time next week, and better still as the weeks go by.

The 'Secret to Happiness', so it turns out, is that there is no secret.

So let's get started.

Making Time to Be Happy

Boxing Day

Here in England we're a little bit odd. And one of our many peculiarities is that Christmas Day, the 25th of December, isn't long enough. Whilst the rest of the world makes more of Christmas Eve, us English folk have declared the 26th of December – the day after Christmas Day – to be 'Boxing Day'.

According to some sources Boxing Day was originally a day when the wealthy would give a boxed gift to their servants. Whether this still happens is something that I haven't the time nor the inclination to find out. But I can tell you that for those of us who *aren't* in servitude, it's another public holiday.

For many years in my family, Boxing Day used to be a re-run of Christmas Day. Sometimes the venue would change but there was always *another* roast turkey dinner, *more* Christmas crackers, *more* party hats, *another* Christmas pud, *more* mince pies and *once again* no one would even touch the Christmas cake. When we were very, very young there even used to be a second round of present giving.

When my wife Kate came along, Boxing Day became 'our' day. We'd get up around midday, open a bottle of champagne, play with our presents from the day before, roast chestnuts in the oven, play silly board games, watch Christmas movies, and eat posh nibbles. It was, quite simply, a fantastic day. Our first Boxing Day together I even ended up asking Kate to marry me. That gives you some idea how good Boxing Day made me feel about life, and there hasn't been a Boxing Day since that hasn't given me a similar inner glow, a similar joy for life.

And I speak with some authority here because in the last five years I've celebrated Boxing Day at least sixty times.

That first Christmas after Kate passed away my mother, concerned for my welfare during the festive season, asked if I'd like to spend Boxing Day with them. It was a generous offer but, call me sentimental, I decided to spend it just as we always had.

I got up late, I opened a bottle of champagne, I sat in bed and browsed my collection of gifts from the previous day. Then I took the Brie from the fridge, a box of posh crackers (the edible kind) and worked my way through the whole lot whilst I sat in front of the telly and watched *The Santa Clause*. A little later I emailed friends I'd been meaning to catch up with, and followed that with a walk down to Old Leigh. I looked out at the boats resting in the mud, and then I went home, wrote down some thoughts, and did some planning.

By the time I went to bed I felt like I'd had a week's holiday, and all I'd done was get out of bed and see how the day unfolded. It was such a good day that I caught myself wishing that Boxing Day happened a little more frequently than once a year, at which point I had the following crazy thought:

Why can't it?

What was to stop me replicating the same structure – or lack of structure – on any other day of the year?

Answer: nothing.

From that day on I decided to have a 'Boxing Day' once a month. Once a month I'd get up with absolutely no plans whatsoever and see how the day unfolded. And that was almost five years ago.

There have been successful Boxing Days (in that I achieve that holiday feeling by the end of the day) and less successful Boxing Days (when I didn't), but there have never been *unsuccessful* Boxing Days (days when I somehow felt more stressed at the end of the day than the beginning). But of all the ideas I've had over the years, Boxing Day has been without a doubt one of the easiest to implement – which is why it's at the start of this book.

The Principles of Boxing Day

From here on, when I refer to Boxing Day, I'm referring
to my Boxing Day, our Boxing Day, the one we are about
to create in your life. Now whether or not you continue to
spend the 26th of December as you have in previous years is
entirely up to you, and whether you want your Boxing Day to
be called 'Boxing Day' or 'Spontaneous Day' or 'Whatever
I Want Day' or something else is equally up to you. I have
one reader, Gaynor (from Wales), who calls it 'WaHay Day',
whilst Heather (down in Texas) calls it 'YOLO (You Only
Live Once) Day'. Amaia (from Spain) calls it something that
I can barely spell let alone pronounce but for the purposes of
this book I'm going to stick with 'Boxing Day', and when I
mention Boxing Day I'm going to assume you realise we're
talking about a day when you give yourself permission to do
whatever you feel like doing, within the realms of possibility,
on the day itself. Let's not get hung up on a name.

Let's cover some basics here: Boxing Day isn't just a
'day off', it's important to get that concept out of your head
immediately. Boxing Day is a day when you get to live totally
in the moment. And why is this important? Because living in
the moment takes a lot less energy!

As adults we expend a huge amount of energy just
juggling the day-to-day. Young children, on the other
hand, don't. They live utterly in the moment and the job of
structuring their day is handled by (hopefully) a responsible
adult. Within the confines of whatever structure is imposed on
them their day is totally driven by what opportunities exist,
right now. They don't *have* to expend any energy on thinking,

and as a result they seem to have bucketfuls of get-up-and-go. You could probably power the whole of Birmingham on half a dozen four-year-olds and a ball pool if you could just keep them in that ball pool long enough.

And four-year-olds never seem to suffer from that Monday morning feeling, they never seem to worry about how they're going to make it through the week, and they never pace themselves. They throw themselves at life, and when they run out of steam, they're done. Have you ever seen the way a four-year-old sleeps? They're so out of it you can pick them up without waking them.

Boxing Day is a little like being a four-year-old for a day. It releases you from thinking about the future or the past. For twenty-four hours everything else is on hold. If you do Boxing Day properly you should feel like you've had a mini holiday – by the end of a Boxing Day you should feel rested, and energised, and happy.

So, let's reiterate how Boxing Day works in one concise sentence:

BOXING DAY IS DRIVEN BY THE MOMENT, THE HEART, AND THE OPPORTUNITY.

Re-read that last sentence because the success of your Boxing Days, should you choose to have them, relies heavily on how well you understand the concept and implement the principles. To boost your chances of success, however, there are some special Boxing Day rules.

Rule Number 1: No Pre-Planning

Everything you do on Boxing Day should be decided on
the day, and determined by what you feel like doing, what's
possible, and what opportunities present themselves. Do not
plan your Boxing Day in advance.

Now you might say to me, 'But I really need to finish
decorating the spare room – taking a day to do that would
be very useful.' Well, fine. If you wake up on Boxing Day
and you really feel like decorating the spare room – if that's
the one thing that would really make your day – then go for
it. Knock yourself out. Personally I hate decorating with a
passion but there have been Boxing Days when I've decided
to 'work', when that's the thing that I want to do more than
any other choices that are available to me. The rule here is
to not, under any circumstances, _plan in advance_ to spend
your Boxing Day up a ladder with a paint brush. If you know
that spare room needs to be decorated then my advice to
you is to set aside another day to do that, and keep Boxing
Day separate. And if decorating the spare room is really that
important, write it down on a piece of paper and come back to
it when we discuss Goals later in this book.

But then you might say to me that your wife / husband /
significant other won't stomach the idea of you taking a day
off 'to do nothing'. To which I would say, you're not going
to do 'nothing'. You're going to do lots. You're just not going
to plan it in advance, and you're not going to let anyone else
determine what you choose to do.

Now having been married I appreciate that this might be
challenging. So, one way to get buy-in from your significant
other is to have a Boxing Day together or, better still,

individual Boxing Days, albeit on the same day. This would avoid a day spent negotiating what the two of you are going to do – or, worse still, one partner dictating or submitting to the other – but I'll leave that for you to decide.

You might also say to me, 'But I'd like to take the kids to this or that attraction and we need to book tickets in advance.' Great. Jot that idea on a piece of paper and we'll come back to it in a few pages' time when we discuss 'Now Lists', but pre-planning a trip to an attraction isn't a valid Boxing Day activity. Waking up on Boxing Day and saying, 'Hey, let's all go to the zoo' – that's fine. Deciding to do it the day before and booking your tickets online – that's not allowed.

And stop stamping your feet on the floor and pulling that face. How old are you? Five? These are the rules and they're there for a reason.

Finally, you might whine, 'But I can't afford all these days off! Mega Corp Ltd only gives me x number of vacation days per year. Blah blah blah.' Oh, for goodness sake! Then allocate one Saturday or Sunday per month to be your Boxing Day! There's no reason to start using up your holiday allocation.

Having said all that, whilst you're not allowed to plan what happens on your Boxing Day, it's still necessary to do some preparation so that Boxing Day actually takes place! Let's not get Planning Boxing Day (a big 'no-no') confused with Planning *to have* a Boxing Day (a big 'yes-yes').

For example, if you're a busy mum with numerous people relying on you to wake them, feed them, clean them, dress them, listen to them, advise them, help them, sympathise with them, transport them … and all the other countless things that come under the Mum job description, standing at the top of the stairs and declaring to the rest of the household that 'today is my Boxing Day', in the vain hope that they'll be able to 'muddle through without you', isn't going to work. You'll probably need to consider at least some of the following:

- What's the best day to have my Boxing Day?
- Should I arrange child care?
- Shall I prepare some microwaveable meals in advance for the family?
- Do I need to warn anyone that I'm 'out for the day'?

You might even need to strike a deal with yourself that whatever you decide to do on Boxing Day – and remember, you can't decide that until the day – will involve 'leaving the house', so as to avoid that temptation to answer the call to Motherly Duty.

Rule Number 2: Book Boxing Day in Advance
This might seem to run contrary to rule number 1, but the only element of Boxing Day that should be pre-planned is deciding when your Boxing Day is going to take place.

If, like me, you use an electronic diary then I recommend you create a monthly Boxing Day appointment. Make it the 26th of each month if you like, especially if you intend to treat the official Boxing Day (the 26th of December) as a Boxing Day. In reality, it doesn't matter when your Boxing Day takes place, so long as it's *regular* and *booked in advance*.

You might have thought that given the spontaneous nature of Boxing Day activities it would make sense for Boxing Day itself to happen spontaneously – wait until you wake up one morning and if you're in a Boxing Day mood, declare that day Boxing Day.

There are two problems with this approach.

Firstly, if you're a workaholic, a 'busy' person, or you work at least five days a week and have commitments most weekends (i.e. someone like me), spontaneity might be something that you struggle with.[4] Therefore a spontaneous Boxing Day would inevitably involve cancelling whatever you had planned. Faced with a lot of last-minute diary shuffling, a task that no one enjoys, it might be easier to be spontaneous another day. Pretty soon Spontaneous Boxing Day would become something that you intend to do, someday, but keep putting off. 'I'll have a Boxing Day tomorrow,' you'll say. 'There's just too much to be done today.'

Secondly, if you're the total opposite of the person above (How do you live? Seriously – how?) then there's an equally good chance that you won't have *any* problems cancelling work, or anything else you had planned. Assuming, of course, that there was anything planned in the first place. Pretty soon you'll be having Boxing Day on a fortnightly, weekly, twice weekly, almost daily basis which will probably have two knock-on effects:

1. The rest of your life won't work, as the stuff that really needs to get done sits in the corner and gathers

---

4 My wife often complained that I wasn't spontaneous enough. In my defence I said that this was nonsense and that I loved being spontaneous, I just preferred to plan it in advance.

dust. Worse still, when you eventually get cut off by
the electricity board you'll blame me and my stupid
Boxing Day idea, and that simply won't do.

2. Boxing Day will lose its potency. Yes, whilst you're
sitting there in the dark, with the bailiffs knocking at
the door, you'll cast your mind back to the day before,
and the day before that, and the day before that, and
realise that Boxing Day just ain't what it used to be –
a week or so ago.

The only way to safeguard against these two scenarios
is to *book Boxing Day in advance*, and make an appointment
with yourself.

But, you might be saying, what if I desperately need a
Boxing Day? Or what if I'm due to have a Boxing Day but
I'm not in the mood, or it's just not convenient? Well, that's
why you need Rule Number 3.

Rule Number 3: You Can Move Boxing Day, But You Can't Cancel It

It's a fact of life that no matter how much you try and
schedule your time, 'stuff happens'. So if today was
supposed to be a Boxing Day but you've just had an echoey
conversation with your best friend who rang you from an
underground sewer after a freak manhole cover incident,
open your diary (planner/calendar/wall chart …), *reschedule*
Boxing Day to another date, then throw a length of rope over
your shoulder, jump in your car and go rescue your friend.

Equally, should you wake up desperately in need of a
Boxing Day, open your diary (planner/calendar/wall chart …)

and see if you can *swap* whatever you had planned for today with your next scheduled Boxing Day.

Believe me, this strategy works well. I've been known to postpone Boxing Days several weeks when Life is throwing everything it can in my direction, and similarly I've been known to have two Boxing Days within a few days of each other if I've deemed it necessary. This rule allows me to respond to the pushes and pulls of daily life whilst still getting an average of 12 Boxing Days a year.

Of course, this rule, and Rule Number 2, are virtually impossible if you don't have a mechanism to manage your time.

Managing Your Time

Time is quite possibly the most valuable commodity you
have. Everything else can be bought with money, and money
itself can be created, found, given, even stolen, but not time.
You have the same number of hours in the day as everyone
else. And whilst you have *some* influence over the number of
those days you might have left, believe me when I tell you
that it doesn't matter how healthy or safety conscious you are,
they can still be snatched away from you at any point.

You've probably heard it said that 'Time is Money'. But
imagine if it was, and the hours and minutes of your life were
somehow controlled by a Universal Bank of Time. What an
austere organisation that would be.

Under their strict account usage terms, the UBT would
actually mandate a compulsory daily *withdrawal* of 24 hours.
The hours would be automatically transferred to you at the
start of each day. However, you could never make a deposit.
You could never put back what you didn't use – and unused
hours would be taxed at 100%. Worse still, the Universal
Bank of Time would steadfastly refuse to issue statements.
There'd be no online banking with the UBT. You couldn't
even get them to give you a balance, so you'd never be sure
how much time you had left.

If real bank accounts worked this way you'd make sure
you spent every penny of your daily withdrawal limit on
something worthwhile. Pretty soon you'd probably start to
plan your spending – you might even keep a book of items
you wanted to spend your money on.

So why don't you do this with your time?

You don't expect to get in your car on Monday morning and have it drive you to work on its own, do you? No. You have to control the darn thing. And it's the same with your life. 'Taking control' comes in many guises, but one of the simplest and most fundamental ways to take control of your life is to manage your time, and to do that:

YOU NEED A DIARY.

When I say 'diary' I mean, of course, a calendar in which you write appointments, not a journal in which you ponder the meaning of life. You might call it your 'planner', or 'schedule', or 'that boring thing that I can't see the point of' – I call it a diary.

Here's what your diary needs to be able to do:
- It needs to be with you (*you*, not your partner), and preferably within arm's reach, at all times
- You need to be able to see a whole week at a glance
- You need to be able to put things in, take things out, and move stuff around, fairly easily

It would also be useful if it could do the following:
- Remind you of upcoming events
- Warn you about public holidays, birthdays, days such as 'Mother's Day', changes to and from British Summer Time[5] etc

---

5   Daylight Saving Time.

These days most people's mobile phones can be set up to do all that and more. But it's not the lack of diary options that stops people from using them, it's the fact that most people don't see the need for one. They're not very sexy. It's all a bit too much like hard work. So let me see if I can sell you some of the benefits of having a diary using real examples from my own life, when I was young and stupid.

Have you ever forgotten someone's birthday? Someone important? How did that feel? Did they give you a hard time about it? Did they get upset? Did they hurl things at you and, in a flurry of tears, accuse you of 'not caring'? That wasn't true, was it – it was simply because your 'current diary system' (i.e. keeping it all in your head) failed you dismally. Am I right? No? Ok, try this …

Have you ever missed an appointment? There you are, sitting on the couch, squinting at the TV, thanking your lucky stars you have an optician's appointment on – oh bugger, it was yesterday. You missed it. And why was that again?

Have you ever parked your car and noticed that the road tax expired last month? And when you went to renew your road tax you discovered that you no longer have a valid MOT (road safety) certificate? Or insurance? Uh huh …

Have you ever arrived at work an hour early – or late – because the clocks changed at the weekend? And you didn't know? Feeling sheepish yet?

Do people phone you up to find out why you haven't turned up to that rehearsal / football match / band practice?

Does it ever seem like you spend your free days doing stuff for other people? Do you ever wonder why you agreed to do that in the first place? Do you ever wish you'd made time for yourself? Have you ever agreed to do something for two different people on the same day? How did it feel when you had to let one of them down?

Do you ever wonder where the time goes? Or how busy people fit it all in? Do you ever wish you could do more – for yourself, get a few things done, make things happen, finish decorating that room, take a day off, go to that concert, take a vacation, spend time with the kids, take a Boxing Day, be happier????

You
need a
diary!

Finding the Right Diary for You

There are some superb diary options out there. I *used* to use
Microsoft Outlook – I hated it with a passion, but it's what
my clients used, and it did the job, albeit in an annoying
Microsoft kinda way.

I'm now using Google Calendar. Compared to Outlook,
Google Calendar is, quite frankly, brilliant. Easy to use, free,
and sophisticated enough that I can share various aspects of
my calendar with trusted friends or work colleagues, and vice
versa. My one and only gripe is that I have to be connected to
the internet to amend it, and more than once I've wished there
was a proper application that I could install on my machine,[6]
similar to the one I have on my iPod.[7]

As you've probably guessed, I'm a diary nerd. And I like
an excuse to play with technology. If you're a technophobe
then an old-fashioned Filofax would work just as well if you
used a pencil and an eraser, and got into the habit of looking
at it on a daily basis. Many, many years ago I used a Franklin
planner and for a while that worked well. Then I moved on –
'upgraded', if you like.

In that respect, diaries are similar to computers. They
don't seem like they're essential, but once you're using one

---

6 Google does have an application you can download that allows you to
view your diary on your computer when you're 'offline' (no internet
connection) – but you can't amend your calendar.

7 CalenGoo is an excellent iPhone App that allows you to view and make
changes to your Google Calendar, even when you're offline – there are
alternatives.

you'll not only wonder how you coped before, but you'll need to upgrade it.

But let's just start with the basics. Let's get you using a diary and managing your time. Let's take action!

Action Points

Throughout this book there are various Action Points. These boxes serve as Stop signs. The idea is that you stop, address the action, and then continue.

Now clearly if you ignore the Action Point – the Stop sign – it's unlikely that you'll be hit by a truck a moment later. Also I'm not going to pursue you through the proceeding pages, flag you down and issue you with a ticket and three points on your Amazon account. That's not going to happen.

Also, I've always been quite enthusiastic about 'ideas'. But whilst I like to collect and share ideas, I fully accept that you have just as much right to ignore them completely. I promise not to get annoyed with you for dismissing any suggestion (and these are only 'suggestions') I throw in your direction, if you promise to forgive me for being a little passionate, or teacher-ish.

That said, I'm assuming you bought this book because something in your head said 'Hey – I *do* want to be happy' and way back on page three, four, something like that, we agreed (well, you read it and I didn't hear you object) that you couldn't achieve this aim without putting a little effort in. So as I'm writing the words, addressing the Action Points is your part of the deal.

With all that in mind, here's the first Action Point of the book:

STOP! ACTION POINT!

Get yourself a diary

Popular options are …
- a paper-based diary (such as a Filofax)
- the calendar on your phone
- Microsoft Outlook
- Google Calendar

Just pick one.

How to Use Your Diary

Hurrah! You have a diary. Fabulous. Now let's start using it.

You might think that's pretty straightforward but you'd be surprised – especially if you're a 'diary newbie' – how easy it is to screw things up. So here's my step-by-step guide:

1) Put ALL your appointments in it. Not just your appointment with your physiotherapist or family planning clinic. Everything. Even the appointments you know you won't forget: your band rehearsals, your evening classes, even WORK. The only possible exception is IF you work a regular five-day week (in which case put the times you're *not* at work in your diary – such as a vacation). If you don't work a five-day week – if you work part-time, or shifts, or you're on a contract – put the work days in. Yes, it looks crowded! Now you know how busy you are.
2) Unless you have another system for this (one that actually works) add all birthdays and anniversaries, and potentially extra reminders a few days ahead of the real event (e.g. you might want an appointment entitled 'It's your wedding anniversary this time next week').[8]
3) Add your own birthday. You'd be surprised how many years I agreed to work on my own bloody birthday!

---

8 An excellent iPhone app that might make this gargantuan task easier is 'Occasions'. Occasions attempts to collate birthdays and anniversaries from the dates in your address book, as well as merging them with people you're friends with on Facebook etc. It'll then warn you about upcoming events. I use this 'warning' to decide whether or not these events get added to my diary.

4) Add public holidays, Easter (remember Easter moves around from one year to the next), Mother's Day, Father's Day, Christmas Day, Boxing Day (the real Boxing Day), Valentine's Day, and both days when they change the damn clocks – in your diary. Links to all these dates are on the website.[9]

5) Delicate one, this one – you may wish to add your menstrual cycle, or the cycle of someone you're close to. I'm just putting the idea out there. Moving on …

6) If your diary has a reminder function, set it to remind you of events and appointments several *days* in advance. Yes, days. Mine is set to ten days (plus the day itself). Birthdays are set to one month. There's no point in getting a reminder about an important birthday or anniversary on the actual day itself – not if you need to get a card and a gift (what d'you mean you always buy the card and gift on the day?)

7) Start checking your diary regularly. How regularly? At least every day (set yourself an alarm if you have to until you get into the habit). You'll be surprised how often you discover an appointment you'd forgotten about. If your diary only allows you to see one day at a time (which is daft – ideally you want to be able to see the whole week in one view) then don't just look at today – have a quick look at tomorrow, and the day after, and the day after that.

---

9 www.howtodoeverythingandbehappy.com. However, if you've elected to use Google Calendar you may be interested to know that you can get it to do this for you by clicking the small down-arrow (next to 'Other Calendars' in the bottom left-hand corner) and then browsing 'Interesting Calendars'.

8) *Before you agree to anything* check your diary again. If the date's free, enter the new appointment. If it's not, decline the appointment, or shuffle stuff around so you can make it.

9) **Do not agree to an appointment if you don't have your diary handy**. Here's how you avoid doing that – you say the following amazing magical phrase:
   'Let me check my diary and get back to you.'
   See how easy that was?

10) Beware people who say, 'What are you doing on …?' It seems like an innocent enough question, and – puffed up with pride in your newly organised life – it'll have you reaching for your diary and revealing to the other person that you're 'free'. Which then makes it virtually impossible to turn down their request to babysit their pet python. Even if you are busy you'll find yourself negotiating over whether what you have planned is more or less important than Percy the Python's happiness and well-being. The appropriate answer to 'What are you doing on …?' is 'Why do you ask?'

11) When agreeing to an appointment check the day before and the day after (so that you don't agree to 'climb a mountain' the day after you 'swim the Channel').

12) When you add an appointment, consider adding supporting appointments. Have you just accepted an invitation to a party? Great. Is it a posh party? Do you need your suit dry cleaned? Will you need a hat? Do you need a present? A card? A partner? Do you need to factor in travel time? Make appointments with yourself on various days before the party to sort out all these things,

along with an appointment (with yourself) to get ready for the party, and to journey to the party itself. Seriously. You'll thank me later. Oh, and book out the day after the party to 'recover'.

13) When you make an appointment remember to add some slack in case it overruns or starts late. Sadly not everyone is as organised as you.

14) Take your diary with you EVERYWHERE. When you leave the house and you check you have your keys, check you have your diary.

15) And finally – make an appointment every month for a Boxing Day.

STOP! ACTION POINT!

Pre-book your Boxing Days

Now that you have your diary, why not create a regular appointment with yourself for Boxing Day? I recommend you start with one a month – maybe on the 26th – always remembering that you can shuffle them about if they're not convenient.

Remember the principle of Boxing Day:

BOXING DAY IS DRIVEN BY THE MOMENT, THE HEART, AND THE OPPORTUNITY

And remember the Boxing Day Rules:
1. No pre-planning what you'll do on the day
2. Book Boxing Day in advance
    (and do whatever preparation's necessary to make sure the day actually happens e.g. arrange childcare, prepare meals etc.)
3. You can move Boxing Day but you can't cancel it

Potential Boxing Day Problems

I can't promise they'll have the same effect on you, but
Boxing Days have had a profound effect on my life; that
simple one day a month has the power to restore my flagging
enthusiasm for life in the way that so many exotic vacations
in the past have utterly failed to.

That said, not every Boxing Day has been a rip-roaring
success. Most of the time that's just because life's like that,
but I've also discovered that Boxing Day has enemies that
like to skulk around in the shadows, waiting for their chance
to mess things up.

Fortunately, my suffering doesn't need to be your
suffering. Here's the spotter's guide to common Boxing Day
problems.

'Excuse Me, But Have You Just Told Me What to Do?'
Perhaps the strangest (for me) feedback I get from readers
are those people who like the idea of Boxing Day, can see the
value of a diary, and would be prepared to take on some of
the other ideas in the book, but can't, because they have an in-
built resistance to being told what to do.

Now personally, so long as I can see the sense in
something and I'm not feeling 'oppressed', I love being told
what to do. It appeals to my very masculine, somewhat nerdy,
love of manuals. Give me a step-by-step guide that gets me
from A to B with the minimum amount of thought and I'm
happy. But if you've spent a lifetime being bossed about,
then I can see how you'd object to me telling you to do X, Y
and Z.

So let's take me out of the equation.

You picked this book up. You decided to read it. You get to decide what you like about it and what you don't. You'll decide what might work, what wouldn't, and what's worth a try. And finally, you'll decide when and how to proceed.

It's all about you.

I'll be over here if you need me.

'Haven't You Re-invented Saturday?'

Not everybody is able to see how a Boxing Day might be a good thing. Some people – let's call them 'young people' – tend to look at me blankly for a moment or two before asking me how a Boxing Day differs from, say, Saturday. Or Sunday. Or virtually any other day of the week when they're not at college. Which seems to be most days.

Before I became the grumpy old sod you see before you now, Saturdays were sacred and followed a very strict routine: I would roll out of bed around midday, and settle down with a bowl of cornflakes in front of _The Chart Show_ before considering whether I should wander down to the town centre to 'mooch about'.

This relaxed state of affairs continued throughout my teens and twenties, and might have continued into my thirties if it hadn't been for the arrival of …

The postman.

If you're in your early twenties you've probably yet to appreciate the sheer amount of admin that awaits you the moment you get a bank account, a loan, a credit card, a car, or move into a place of your own. Suddenly there's a mountain of paperwork to be addressed, most of it hidden amongst an even bigger mountain of junk from people trying to sell you stuff. And whilst you can (as I did) leave this stuff on the side in the hope that it'll kind of sort itself out, I don't recommend it. Handing over your money to these organisations is only part of the payment required – the remainder is due in time, sorting out all manner of insurances, car repair bills, and taxes of numerous flavours. And that's assuming that you never miss a payment, your boiler never packs up, and the Gas Board doesn't decide to change your supplier without your knowledge. If you manage to juggle all this nonsense without surrendering the occasional Saturday I take my hat off to you. Personally I'd developed a morbid fear of 'post' by the time I was thirty.

Of course you might, as many people do, assume that there's strength in numbers, and choose to combine forces with another. And whilst there are most definitely perks to giving up your single life, it's only a matter of time before your entire weekend is given over to ferrying the kids around, climbing a ladder with a paintbrush in your hand, or wandering the aisles of Ikea trying to find the damn exit.

When that happens, you might consider booking yourself a Boxing Day.

Not Knowing What to Do
Ideally here's how Boxing Day should work: you wake up, you ask yourself what you fancy doing at that precise moment, then you go and do that thing. And when you've done that, or you've had enough of whatever it is, you go and do something else. Easy?

Not necessarily.

Once you've decided (in advance) when your Boxing Day will be, gremlins immediately take up residence under your bed, ready to thwart you.

The first gremlin is 'your usual daily routine'. Unless you begin Boxing Day right away it's incredibly easy to start the day pretty much as every other and before you know it you're checking emails, opening post and oh, the laundry basket's looking a little full, I'll just put on a load of washing.

The second is a 'general lack of inspiration'. There you are. Sitting in bed. Ready for the Boxing Day euphoria to kick in just as soon as you can decide what it is that you'd like to do … and you just can't think of anything.

I've been there.

Here then are some top tips should you find yourself in a similar situation:

1) *Start Boxing Day from the moment you open your eyes* – Try and break from your normal daily routine from the moment you wake up. A couple of times I've come downstairs and as I've reached for the milk in the fridge I've seen those eggs, sitting there, quietly doing nothing, and thought to myself – sod it – let's cook breakfast. And other times, as I opened the cupboard to take out the Weetabix, I've noticed a kilo bag of oats and thought to myself, 'You know, what I really fancy right now are flapjacks.'

2) *Perform the Boxing Day Dance* – Flushed with the success of the first Boxing Day (which you'll remember was an accident) I was quite excited when, having made an appointment with myself, it was time to have the

second one. I was so excited that I danced round the flat in my dressing gown making up a silly Boxing Day song as I went, much to the bemusement of my cat. Strange thing is, though, I've since found that if I'm having a Boxing Day which feels a little flat, a few bars of my Boxing Day song will be all I need to get the Boxing Day juices flowing. (No you can't hear my Boxing Day song – make up your own!)

3) *Do the first thing that comes to mind* – Sometimes it's difficult to decide what to do with your Boxing Day because you're over-thinking it. If you're struggling to feel inspired, stop, and ask yourself: 'What do I want to do RIGHT NOW?' The thing that comes to mind, usually before you've even finished the sentence, is very possibly the thing you should do. It doesn't matter how silly it may seem, or how simple – if it can be done, now, and you like the idea – do it!

4) *You can work* – Working on Boxing Day is a completely legitimate exercise if that's what you really want to do. And let's broaden the definition of work to include any activity that you might not consider typically 'fun'. Decorating, for instance. Balancing your cheque book. Filling out an application form. Don't put yourself under pressure to fill your Boxing Day with 'fun' activities. If it's what you want to do (*want* to do – not *need* to do) then it's a legitimate Boxing Day activity. For instance, I am writing this paragraph on a Boxing Day! That's the absolute truth, and I can honestly say that right now, given the moment, the opportunities available to me, and how I feel, writing this is what I *really* want to do. (That said, I

drove an hour and a half to Cambridge, and found myself
the trendiest independent coffee shop to act as my writing
venue. You get the idea.)

5) *Make a list* – Pre-planning Boxing Day is <u>utterly</u>
forbidden, but if you're a planner at heart (as I am),
there's nothing to say you can't do a little brainstorming
at the start of the day. If I don't wake up and feel instantly
inspired I often grab a piece of paper (rather than sit at
my computer) and jot down ideas – things that I *could*
do. I try and write my ideas all over the page and at weird
angles so that it's as un-list-like as possible (otherwise
I might be tempted to start at the top and work through
the items). And then, when I've finished brainstorming,
quite often I'll toss the list to one side and do something
entirely different.

6) *You can be dull* – If you want to do nothing but sit on the
sofa and watch TV, or go back to bed, or read a magazine
cover to cover, or play computer games, that's perfectly
acceptable. If it's been a while since your last Boxing Day
(perhaps you had to postpone it) then maybe this is the
first opportunity you've had in a while to rest. So do it.
Rest. However, I encourage you to rest *with gusto* – if you
want to go back to bed, put your PJs back on, close the
curtains, put on some soothing music, maybe download
some 'ocean sounds' to your iPod, sprinkle lavender on
your pillow – really go for it! If you want to watch TV,
grab some snacks, then sit down and watch an entire
season of *Lost*, or *24*, or *Gilmore Girls*, or *Doctor Who*, or
whatever floats your boat.

Towards the back of this book, under the section 'Putting It All Together', you'll find an example of what a typical Boxing Day looks like (for me).

Pre-Planning Your Boxing Day
No, no, no, no, and a thousand times no!

People Ambush Your Boxing Day
'What you up to today?' asks a friend.

'I'm having a Boxing Day,' you reply.

That's not what they'll hear, of course. Somehow the words will get scrambled somewhere between leaving your mouth and entering their ears, and what they'll hear is: 'I'm doing nothing.'

Which is why they suddenly invite themselves over, or ask if you'd like to help them paint their lounge, out of some misguided notion that they're somehow enhancing your day and you'd otherwise be sitting there bored out of your mind.

Bang goes Boxing Day.

It's a little like finding a tranquil picturesque location, then sitting down to do a watercolour painting, only to have the person next to you reach over and start filling in bits you haven't done yet. But can you tell them this? No. Of course not.

There's only one solution to this problem. And it's a matter of 'prevention' rather than 'cure' – keep your Boxing Day SECRET, and when asked what you're up, do not tell people (including friends – especially friends!) that you're having a Boxing Day, tell them something else!

Spending Boxing Days with Other People

Continuing the theme, whilst Boxing Day is all about *you*, and doing the things that you want to do, you don't *have* to spend it on your own. Feel free to call up a pal and do something together if that's what you want – just be prepared for the possibility that they:

1. might not be able to drop everything at a moment's notice, thereby scuppering your plans, or
2. having dropped everything they understandably want a say in the day's activities, thereby compromising the true spirit of Boxing Day.

Boxing Days If You're in a Relationship

Struggling to have a Boxing Day inside the confines of a relationship? Then try this.

Reader Helen and her husband created Be Nice to Helen Days, and Be Nice to Les Days (Les being her husband, not some random person). On your day you're allowed to determine what happens and the other person has to go along with it – no arguments.

I could see how that could work. Just stay true to yourself and try not to fall into the trap of picking things that the two of you will like, or worse, that the other person will like and you don't. In fact, I'd go as far to say drag your other half to that romantic comedy, or take your partner to that football match, and if you are the other party, go with it – your day will come.

Boxing Days If You're a Parent

Reader Jane dropped me a line:

'I think I've figured out something that may help in terms of "how Mums can do a Boxing Day". You may need to relax the "rules". The thing is, there is always so much to do around the house and for the kids/husband/etc.

'If I had planned a bit more beforehand (e.g. booked a massage, picked a film to go and see, arranged to meet a friend for lunch, booked a table to eat alone, etc) then I might have had more of a successful BD. However, because (the rules state) you're not "allowed" to think about what you're doing in advance, I ended up doing a whole load of chores and things that needed doing around the house. Which was fine, but not really the rest a 36-week pregnant woman with a one-year-old needed!

'I suggest that childcare is arranged, even if it's just for half a day with Grandparents, and then you allow Mums to book one thing to do (or plan one thing to do) outside of the house. This would remove the temptation to go ahead and get on with chores, etc.

'A Mum's (and I'm sure a Dad's!) lot is a busy one and there is, like I say, always so much to do that it's hard to put oneself first, especially if you have that rare commodity of free time. The first thing that comes to mind is something along the lines of "Thank goodness! Now I can get that big pile of ironing done, weed the garden, cook for the freezer, etc."'

My gut reaction to Jane's email was to point out that there's a huge difference between pre-planning (what you're going to do on Boxing Day) and preparing (doing whatever's necessary so that a Boxing Day is possible). Pre-planning is bad. Preparing, on the other hand, is very, very good. Necessary even.

However, hot on the heels of Jane's email, readers Kirsty and Alison contacted me with very similar thoughts! It seems it's just too darn difficult to be spontaneous on a Boxing Day if you're a mum – other stuff always gets in the way. Clearly I'm out of my depth here.

So I called in the Big Guns and emailed Keris Stainton[10] – author, journalist, fan of this book and (most importantly) *Busy Mum of two*. I put the Busy Mum vs Boxing Day conundrum to her, reserved several pages in this chapter for her words of wisdom, and waited. If anyone would know the answer it would be Keris. Why, she'd probably end up writing a blog post or an article about it.[11] Fabulous!

Three weeks later (I told you she was busy) I got her response.

She was, to use her own words, 'flummoxed' – unable to see how being a busy parent is so different from being a busy anything else. She went on to say:

'If the FIRST thing you think of when you get up on Boxing Day is "Thank goodness – now I can get that big pile of ironing done, weed the garden, cook for the freezer, etc", then, well, you REALLY need a Boxing Day!'

If any of this rings true for you then let me just say this: go for it. And if 'going for it' means you need to have one thing pre-arranged, or you have to have a rule that says Boxing Day takes place off-site, or you limit Boxing Day to

10   www.keris-stainton.com
11   She blogs on parenting over at parentdish.co.uk. Interesting stuff.

the hours between dropping the kids off and picking them back up again, or Boxing Day is something you do with another Busy Parent – if that 'fixes' Boxing Day and makes it work for you – *then you have my blessing*! I am not going to stand in your way. I'm just pleased that you're finally taking time out for yourself.

If you're a parent and have any thoughts on the challenges of Boxing Day, feel free to share them on the website or on the Facebook page.[12]

Too Many Boxing Days – Not Enough Boxing Days
So if one Boxing Day a month can work such magic, surely two Boxing Days a month would be twice as good, right?

Apparently not.

Believe me, I've tried.

For reasons that I've never really understood, too many Boxing Days actually reduces their effectiveness. They cease to be 'special' – and being 'special' is possibly what makes them work so well.

One Boxing Day a month seems just about right. Two just doesn't work.

However, this said, there's a chance that it might be different for different people. Unfortunately, even though I invented Boxing Day (or re-invented it ... whatever...) I've only myself to experiment on. Therefore I encourage you to conduct your own experiments. If you feel you need more, squeeze an extra one in and see if it works. If on the other hand your Boxing Days start to feel more like a boring

---

12   www.facebook.com/howtodoeverythingandbehappy

Sunday afternoon than a week in a five-star hotel, or if you
end up with a Boxing Day backlog (i.e. you postpone so
many that you actually start to have more than one 'in the
bank') well, chances are you're having too many.

Too Busy to Have a Boxing Day
In stark contrast to those under the age of twenty-five there
are those people who are utterly convinced that they couldn't
possibly take one day out a month for themselves. They're
just too darn busy.

In my experience there are two types of 'I don't have the
time {for Boxing Day}' people – those that don't have the
time, and those that *think* they don't have the time. Let's find
out which type you are.

Answer this simple two-part question:

DO YOU HAVE AN APPOINTMENT DIARY

AND

DO YOU USE IT?

If you haven't answered yes to both parts, chances are
you're one of the people who only *think* that they're busy.
What you're calling 'busy' is in fact 'chaos'.

I'm not kidding about this: diaries really are *that*
important. Where were you when we covered this a few pages
back?

Go get a diary, and start using it.

Meanwhile, let's have a look at what the rest of you are
spending your time on.

Hmmm. I see.

Well, you're right. You do indeed appear to have a very busy schedule. Every single moment is indeed booked out for something. That'll be why you have that smug 'told you so' look on your face that's just crying out for a smack.

But wait – what's this appointment here? Every Sunday?

'That's when I go to see my mother,' you say.

'Every Sunday?'

'Well, yes.'

'Could you not skip it one week?'

'Not really.'

'Why?'

'Because she expects me!'

'So tell her you can't make it one week!'

'I couldn't do that,' you say.

'Why not?'

'Because she's my mother.'

'Ok, but what about this Sunday? This Sunday you're not seeing your mother. This says "work".'

'Well yes,' you reply. 'There's this big project we're finishing up, and my boss really needs me – and besides, it's overtime …'

'So it's ok to cancel your mother if there's overtime up for grabs?'

'Well, we're really busy right now …'

'And your mother's ok with that?'

'Well, it's work – it's important.'

'And you're not important?'

'Sorry?'

'I said: "You're not important?"'

'Well, of course I am, I suppose …'

'You suppose?'

'Look, I can't cancel my mother, not to spend a day by myself ...'

'Because you're not important?'

'Well, er ...'

'Well?'

It's not that you're too busy, it's that you're putting everyone and everything before you and your happiness! You have, in effect, trained yourself – yes, *trained yourself* – to believe that when it comes to <u>your</u> time, and <u>your</u> life, everyone else gets to say how you spend it.

You *need* to stop that.

Of course, that's easier said than done. From birth we're encouraged by others to take on that 'training'. Eventually we might even convince ourselves that these habits of selflessness/martyrdom/workaholism are a good thing. We say to ourselves, 'I must be a good person, I put everyone else first – yay me.' Those that don't adopt a similar saintly attitude – and you can probably think of someone off the top of your head – can, on occasion, come across as a little self-centred or selfish. Maybe more than a little. And maybe not as occasionally as you'd like. Thank God you're not like that.

I bet they're happier, though.

Now I'm not suggesting for one minute that you become like them, but accepting that you've created a habit of surrendering your time without question, and becoming aware of that habit, will give you the opportunity to say 'no' and gradually regain control of your life. It'll feel uncomfortable at first. It may even feel wrong. At some point you'll upset someone. Maybe several someones. And that'll make you feel guilty. But these things will pass. With practice it'll become easier – it'll start to make sense – and the people around, those that care about you, will, eventually, adjust to the 'new you'.

So – let's start now – go tell your mother that you won't make it next week, or your boss that you can't come in on Sunday.

People Who REALLY Don't Have Enough Time for Boxing Day
'Dear Mr Jones,

I recently purchased your book "How to Do Everything and Be Happy" – and today I stopped reading it.

How dare you suggest that I am not really busy? There are those amongst us who are lucky if we can claw back five minutes from the day to spend doing what we want!

I am a single mother with two children and an elderly sick relative who needs my constant attention. When my day finally ends I sometimes spend a few minutes reading when I should probably be sleeping. This is the only time I get to myself, and I do not appreciate being told by you, a single man, that I'm not really busy.

You're right – I don't own a diary, but this is because I don't need a diary – every single day is exactly the same! And yes, you're right, everybody else does get to say how I spend my time – everybody else, as you quite rightly said, does come before me and my happiness. I don't like it, but that's how the world is, so you can take your book and shove it somewhere uncomfortable.

Yours sincerely,

Ms Fictitious (but nonetheless Very Cross) Person'

'Dear Ms Very Cross Person,

You're right.

Please accept my apologies if this book has offended you in any way. I don't have all the answers. I truly wish I did. And the answers that I do have aren't necessarily easy to achieve, or right for everyone.

I've never been in your situation where so many people you care about are relying on you to supply their most basic of needs. I can only imagine how challenging that must be.

I do know, however, that raising kids isn't just about getting the "must dos" out of the way – if you're anything like my sister or the other mums I've spoken to, then as well as making sure they're clothed and fed, you probably want to do whatever you can to enable your children to pursue their own activities and dreams whenever possible. For years my mother ferried me to and from cubs, scouts, drama club, youth club, swimming club ... the list goes on.

Of all these activities swimming was a favourite. By the time I was in my early teens I was working on my survival badges. I'd spend evenings jumping in and out of swimming pools, fully clothed, picking up bricks from the bottom of the pool and taking it in turns to "rescue" my fellow swimming club members. When the evening ended I'd present my mother with a bag full of sopping wet clothes without a second thought as to what she was going to do with them.

Whilst I was utterly guilty of taking my mother for granted, I was nonetheless learning some important skills. And though I've never had to rescue bricks or people, or inflate my trouser bottoms into a floatation device, or give anyone the kiss of life, there is one swimming survival concept that has stayed with me my whole life. We were always taught that when rescuing a drowning person, if the drownee begins to thrash or struggle, such that your attempts at rescue are being compromised, you need to push them away – just for a moment – just until you regain control, and you're able to resume your rescue.

Whilst finding an entire day to call your own might be impossible right now, it is, nonetheless, vital to look after yourself. I sincerely believe you need to find a way to push "them" away – just for a few moments – and regain control of your life. Not just for your own sanity, but because you'll be no use to them if you drown.

Take care
Sincerely
Peter Jones'

Advanced Boxing Day – Extra Tips!

So you recently had a Boxing Day. You obeyed all the rules, took all the advice on the previous few pages – and yet somehow it *still* didn't rock your world. Maybe it was a little dull.

That can happen.

It's happened to me.

In fact the more Boxing Days I had, the more it happened. And when I came to analyse it (because sadly that's the sort of thing I do) I came to the conclusion that Boxing Day might need some tweaking.

Here are a couple of new ideas that I've been experimenting with since the first edition of this book and are really working for me.

Avoid Hedonistic Habituation

Once you've had a few Boxing Days it becomes surprisingly difficult to keep your Boxing Days totally spontaneous. I got into a bad habit of always having a bottle of champagne, and always making a truck load of flapjacks. Not only was this a tad expensive, but after a while Boxing Day started to lose its magical powers.

What I hadn't realised at the time was that I was experiencing something that scientists refer to as 'Hedonistic Habituation'. Regardless of how pleasurable an activity is, much of its pleasure is actually derived from its 'newness'. So whilst I thought I was relying on activities that had worked on previous Boxing Days, I had, in fact, got myself into a boozy, flapjacky rut.

This seems so obvious now. Though it's also a little annoying. It means that even when I eventually get to emulate my hero Julio Casi Amoreo,[13] my days spent sitting around the pool of my villa in southern Italy, admiring my scantily clad 'friends', will get progressively less and less pleasurable the more familiar it becomes.

Fortunately there's an antidote:

DO SOMETHING NEW

To avoid Hedonistic Habituation, when your Boxing Day arrives try to do at least one 'new thing', and if possible, make that the first thing you do.

Now come on.

Don't be like that.

I know how hard that sounds and I realise I've made Boxing Day a whole lot more difficult. Not only have you got to pre-book Boxing Day, arrange for baby-sitters and the like, tell friends and family that you're doing something else, *and* avoid the temptation to plan something for the day, but when the day actually arrives you've somehow got to conjure a new activity out of thin air? Just what kind of self-help book is this?! But bear with me for a moment, because I have two simple techniques that will enable you to do just that.

---

13   See earlier in the book under Work / Life Balance.

Tweak Previous Activities

An astonishingly simple way of coming up with new Boxing Day activities is to think back to past Boxing Days and things you did that were a real hit, and tweak them!

Take me, for example. Last Boxing Day, rather than reach for a kilo of oats and a tin of golden syrup, I decided to make chocolate brownies. Have I ever made chocolate brownies before? No. Were they any good? Mmmm … not really.[14] Did I enjoy myself? Absolutely.

So if you've got into the habit of going to the gym on your Boxing Days, try a different exercise class, or a different gym. If you find you always go fishing, try a different lake or river. If you find yourself painting watercolours, experiment with charcoal sticks or oil pastels. If you usually end up on the sofa watching rom-coms, download a rom-com to your e-reader. Or go to the cinema. Or watch an action movie instead. You get the general idea.

The interesting thing is that most activities only require the smallest bit of tweaking in order to activate that part of your brain that gets enjoyment out of 'the new'. And once it's activated it's amazing how little effort the rest of the day needs to be a success.

Let me know how you get on.

---

14 Top tip: when making chocolate brownies remember to add the chocolate and the cocoa powder. It makes all the difference.

Potential Boxing Day Activities List

A second way to ensure that you can always think of something new is to keep a 'Potential Boxing Day Activities List'.

As you progress through this book you'll discover that I'm a bit of a list maniac. 'Lists' are my solution to everything. And when it comes to potential Boxing Day activities it really works. Where and how you keep your list is entirely up to you, but personally I like to keep a 'notepad' document on my computer's desktop so that I can open the list, add to it, save it, and close it again, all within a few seconds. You might be able to keep a list on your phone. Or in the back of your Filofax. Or in a small notepad in your handbag. But whatever you do, it's important that the list is usually close to hand so that when inspiration strikes you can add to the list right away.

Remember too that to be true Boxing Day potentials, all the activities on the list must be things that require no pre-planning. The only time you're going to consult this list is either when you add to it, or when you bound out of bed on Boxing Day morning.

I can't claim 100% credit for the Potential Boxing Day list. Within days of me mulling the concept over in my mind, reader Emma posted a comment on the How to Do Everything and Be Happy blog suggesting much the same thing.

On her list of Potential Boxing Day ideas were the following:

- Get the tattoo I've been wanting for a while
- Visit the zoo/cinema/theatre
- Get a massage/manicure
- Go shopping at Manchester/Newcastle or anywhere within a three-hour radius
- Go walking/gym/swimming
- Bake something
- Horse riding

Emma says that having the list there meant that she actually got excited about the idea of Boxing Day – which can only be a good thing.

Timing

Like good comedy, the success of your Boxing Day might rely heavily upon timing.

Though I don't make it a hard and fast rule, I have been known to move Boxing Day to avoid bad weather, or times when I'm particularly tired. And whilst you'd think that a Boxing Day might be a good way to lift your spirits if you're feeling a bit low, personally I've found the complete opposite is true.

Boxing Day seems to have the ability to make good days even better – but also bad days significantly worse.

You'll probably already know if there are certain times of the month when a Boxing Day might be doomed to failure. I suspect it's a very personal thing, but I have readers who avoid the following times of the month:

- 'The end of the month – I get paid at the start!'

- 'My menstrual cycle – there's nothing worse than feeling yuk on a Boxing Day.'
- 'A week or so after a full moon – when the moon is waning.'

Cut Yourself Some Slack!

Though it pains me to admit it, despite all the rules, tips and advice I've given you, I can't guarantee that Boxing Day will work each and every time. Occasionally, as I said a little earlier, you're bound to have a duff one.

It took me a long time to accept this fact, but I've learned that when this happens it's best just to shrug, and move on. For when it comes to creating happiness, whilst Boxing Days are great, they're not the whole answer.

Well, of course they're not!

If they were then this would be the end of the book! And it's just the beginning. Hold on to your hats, people, because we've just gotten started!

Doing Those Things You Always Wanted to Do

So how do you feel? Happier? How's Boxing Day working out for you? What did you decide to call it in the end?

Of course I realise that you've probably only just turned the page and you're yet to make your first Boxing Day appointment, let alone enjoy the experience, but I hope at the very least you're enjoying the book. You're still reading it – I'll take that as a good sign.

Onwards then.

Do you like movies?

The Bucket List

In 2007 Morgan Freeman and Jack Nicholson starred in a film called *The Bucket List*. These two great actors play terminally ill gentlemen who share a hospital room. With only weeks to live, the two characters write a list of things they want to experience before they 'kick the bucket' – they call it their 'bucket list' – and set about trying to complete each one.

Here's the list they came up with:

- Witness something truly majestic
- Help a complete stranger for the good
- Laugh till I cry
- Drive a Shelby Mustang
- Kiss the most beautiful girl in the world

- Get a tattoo
- Skydiving
- Visit Stonehenge
- Spend a week at the Louvre
- See Rome
- Dinner at La Chèvre d'Or, Eze
- See the Pyramids
- Get back in touch
- Visit the Taj Mahal
- Hong Kong
- Victoria Falls
- Go on a safari
- Drive a motorcycle on the Great Wall of China
- Sit on the Great Egyptian Pyramids
- Find the joy in your life

It's a great movie. And it really makes you think: what would you do if someone gave you only six weeks to live?

Personally, if someone gave me six weeks to live I'd be a basket case by the end of the first afternoon! Assuming I could get my head round the shocking news, drawing up that list of experiences for my *final six weeks* would be like telling myself a thousand times over that I'd wasted the previous X number of years. And completing the items on my list would only serve to remind me of my dwindling mortality.

Basically, it's the stuff of nightmares.

I'd much rather be in a position whereby, having been given the awful news, I could take solace in the fact that I'd *already* had a life full of exciting, fun and interesting experiences. And were someone to hand me a big yellow legal pad and a pen (as they do in the movie) I'd much rather struggle to think of anything I hadn't already experienced at some point in my life.

Of course, given that most of us have very little idea how many days we actually have left, for the above to be true I'd have to do something about it, well … today! Now! I'd have to grab a pen (you do have one handy, don't you?) and start jotting down all those things that I want to experience, and then damn well set about doing them as soon as possible.

So guess what this section of the book's all about?

Creating a 'Live Life Now' List

Firstly, let's dispense with the term Bucket List. That's not what we're creating here. We don't want to be sitting in a hospital bed thinking of all the things we never did. What we want is to Live Life Now. So that's what we're going to call it. A 'Live Life Now' list – or a 'Now List' for short.

Writing a Now List is pretty straightforward. If you're a bit of a traditionalist – 'retro' as the cool kids call it – take out a sheet of paper, write Now List at the top, then put it somewhere you'll find it again without a lot of searching.

If you're a little more tech savvy, I encourage you to create an empty document on your computer and/or phone and save it as 'Now List'.

Notice that all we're doing here is creating a *blank* document, and labelling it. If you can already think of items you want on your Now List then go ahead and write them down, but it's just as likely that you can't think of anything, or the one or two items you have seem a little lame. That's because all the things that *should* make your list are locked within your memory. They're the moments when you declared – either out loud or in your head – 'I've always wanted to do that,' right before you forgot all about it.

That's not going to happen again.

Next time someone tells you that they've just come back from a six-month round the world trip, or someone asks you to sponsor them in the London Marathon, or you drive past that building you've always wanted to go inside, or your favourite band is advertising their next world tour, or a hot-air balloon floats over your house – and you find yourself thinking, 'Wow – I'd really love to …' – THAT'S the moment you're going to jot down a reminder and add that item to your Now List.

It's important then to *create an empty list now*, ready and waiting for your next 'I'd really love to do that' moment. Trust me – don't wait until you have a Now List item. That doesn't seem to work. And how do I know that? Because that's exactly what I did! But once the list had been created ideas started coming thick and fast.

Save yourself some time – create the Now List, now.

Stop! Action Point!

Create an empty Now List.

Whether you choose to maintain an electronic list, or a paper one, go and create your Now List now, ready for the next time you say 'I'd really love to …'

Deciding What's On the List

Anything you write on your list should be an answer to the following question:

**WHAT WOULD I LIKE TO EXPERIENCE
(BEFORE I DIE)?**

The key word there is *experience*. This isn't some sort of to-do list of things you have to get done before you check out. So items like 'make sure the kids are taken care of', or 'pay off the mortgage', or 'give my stash of *Doctor Who* comics to my nephew' have no place on your Now List.

Similarly this isn't a list of goals or personal milestones. So whilst you might want to 'write a best-selling novel', or 'learn to play the saxophone', or 'get married', or 'patch things up with my Aunt', all before you run out of days, they're a little bigger than mere experiences. They're all fabulous – and if any of these things resonate with you then you should definitely consider doing them, but – without wanting to get ahead of ourselves – jot them down and we'll come back to them in the next section.

Your Now List should be made up of experiences that theoretically you could do right now, if you were free, had the money, and you could hop back in time to do some preparation. In other words, your Now List is for all those things you couldn't do on a Boxing Day because they require some pre-planning and forethought.

So for example, here's my Now List:

- Take a narrow boat through Birmingham
- Go on boat trips (see my house from the Estuary)
- Get close to lemurs
- Get close to dolphins
- Make Mum's Treacle Tart
- Visit the Minack Theatre
- Have dinner with Imogen Heap
- Get tickets to her Albert Hall gig
- Work with Steven Moffat
- Rome!
- Go back to Sorrento
- Visit Hong Kong
- Go round the world (in a westerly direction)
- Visit the Cook Islands
- Play a part in *The Importance of Being Earnest*

Now if, having peeked at my list, you're already getting ideas or you want to pinch some of mine, well what are you reading this for? Go – add those items to your list! Do it now!

Categorising Your Now List

The problem with the underlying Now List question ('What would you like to experience before you die?') is that it's totally overwhelming. It's a little like when someone asks you to tell them a joke – every joke you've ever heard momentarily disappears from your head. Even really funny people struggle to think of anything to say.[15]

But if we break the 'before you die' question into sub-questions, they become 'smaller', and easier to answer.

For instance, aside from the obvious 'What places would you like to visit? Are there any bands you'd like to hear play? Or plays you'd like to see or be in?' – effectively what we're doing here is breaking your Now List into categories which will help to generate ideas AND make the list easier to manage.

Two of my favourite categories are:

- Distant dreams (for items that seem utterly ludicrous right now – e.g. walk on the moon)
- Food I'd really like to try

These are only suggestions. If you're not a foodie, forget about the food category. If you're a sporty person, or a musical person, you might like to create categories for those. It really doesn't matter. But the more categories your Now List has, the easier it gets to think of items you want on it.

---

15 Here's a good one: two fish in a tank, one says to the other, 'How d'you drive this thing?'

With categories, my list looks like this:

Time sensitive
- Take a narrow boat through Birmingham
- Visit the Minack Theatre
- See Imogen Heap at the Albert Hall
- Go to a Bill Bailey gig

Animal magic
- Get close to lemurs
- Get close to big cats
- Get close to dolphins

Places I'd like to visit
- Rome!
- Go back to Sorrento
- Visit Hong Kong
- Go round the world (in a westerly direction)
- Visit the Cook Islands

Distant dreams
- Have dinner with Imogen Heap
- Work with Steven Moffat
- And Richard Curtis

Food I'd really like to try
- Make Mum's Treacle Tart
- Try deep fried crickets or some other insect (from the night-time food market in Beijing)

Other
- Go on boat trips (see my house from the Estuary)
- Play a part in *The Importance of Being Earnest*

'Time Sensitive' is a useful category to have. It forces you to think of all the things you'd like to do which are anchored to a particular point in history or season. The 2016 Olympics, for instance; I'm pretty sure it'll be over by 2017. And a narrow boat holiday through the centre of Birmingham in the middle of January might be a little grim. That's definitely a summer activity.

Notice how a few new items have found their way onto my list. The Treacle Tart item looked quite lonely sitting on its own in the food category, which is when I remembered something else that I've always wanted to eat – deep fried crickets! That's the power of categories.

Remember, your Now List items don't have to be hugely impressive. My brother turned his nose up when he discovered that seeing Imogen Heap is on my list. 'That,' he said, 'is not really a Now List item.' Which brings me to a very, very important point:

IT'S **<u>YOUR</u>** LIST.

It's your happiness we're planning here. If other people don't like the items on your list tell them to make their own! Seeing Imogen Heap is a big deal for me. Therefore it makes the list. Some people absolutely love movies. Those folks might start creating a list of films they must see 'before they die' and who are we to tell them that they can't do that?

My friend Tina has a cupboard full of board games that she could never coax any of her family to sit down and play. Consequently, 'organise a games evening' went on her Now List.[16]

Finally, a word about the 'other' category. Generally speaking I'm not a big fan of categories called 'other' or 'miscellaneous'. They very quickly become a dumping ground for items that should have a category of their own – but when it comes to Now Lists this can be a good thing. It'll encourage your imagination to dream up stuff that doesn't fit under the other categories you've created. As soon as your 'other' category has two or more items that look like they could team up and form a category of their own, go ahead and do that.

Time, I think, for some action:

---

16 It took place back in February. A hilarious evening! I'm thinking of stealing the idea and putting it on my list.

Stop! Action Point!

Create Now List categories

Aside from the obvious 'places you'd like to visit' category, and an 'other' category, think of categories that'll help you generate ideas for your Now List. You might use some or all of the following:

Places I'd like to visit
Food I'd like to try
People I'd like to meet
Distant dreams
Animal magic
Bands I'd like to see
Books I really want to read
Sports I want to master
Things to do as a couple or *Me & The Lads / Girls*
Time sensitive
Other

Making Your Now List 'Happen'

So you have your Now List – what now?

This might seem like a daft question. Obviously the answer is 'start working through it' – but, if you're like me, you might go for the popular second choice: 'put it in a drawer (virtual or otherwise) and ignore it.'

That's what I did with my list for the first year. Which meant that from the very first moment I decided to create a Now List, to the day I started to do something about it was *eighteen months*. A year and a half of my life had rolled by when I could have visited several amazing places or eaten many strange and wonderful things.

So, you might ask, why did it take me so long?

It's hard to say. Maybe I took a look at the list and realised that most of the items were going to take some planning, or money, or time, or something else I didn't have at that exact moment.

Maybe I was afraid – after all, I hate travelling on my own and my list does have quite a few places that I'd like to visit. But not on my own.

Maybe I had a deep-rooted psychological desire to maintain the status quo of my life and the Now List threatened that by representing *change*. Do the items on my Now List and I might, for a moment, *feel happier*. Once happier, I might be driven to change more things in my life. Where would it all end?!

Who knows? Who cares! The point is, the list was locked away and as such it was a waste. A waste of paper, a waste of time, and a waste of potential happiness.

Which is why I created Now List Day.

Now List Day

Welcome to your Now List Day. A day, once a month, where one of two things will happen:

1. You will enjoy an item on your Now List, or
2. You will work through your Now List and take whatever actions necessary to make your Now List items a reality.

So first, go back to your diary (you do have a diary, don't you? Let's not get started on that again ...) and book out one day a month for a Now List Day.

Those of you who struggled to find one day a month for Boxing Day will be bouncing off the walls right now at the thought of clawing back a few hours to spend on your Now List, so I'll cut you a deal: if you really can't find a whole day then allocate a couple of Now List evenings, mornings, or lunchtimes. Whatever works for you. Just regular slots. Now clearly it's going to be difficult to climb Mount Everest during your lunch hour, or visit The Seven Wonders of the World, or play with Eric Clapton at Wembley, or whatever you have on your list, but you can at least do some planning and research. Find someone who's planning to climb Everest, purchase a round trip Seven Wonders of the World ticket, or email Mr Clapton's agent.

Towards the back of this book, under the section 'Putting It All Together', you'll find an example of what a typical Now List (planning) Day looks like (for me).

Like Boxing Day, Now List Day has rules to help you make it a success:

1. Now List Days/slots can be moved, but not cancelled
2. Only two things happen on a Now List Day –
   a. you're either doing something on the list so that you can check it off, or
   b. you're planning/researching/booking items on your list for sometime in the future.

Ready to start turning those Now List ideas into memories?

STOP! ACTION POINT!

Book your Now List Days into your diary

Or Now List lunchtimes.
Breakfasts.
Evenings.
Whatever works for you.

The Trophy Board

Andy Warhol, so it's said, never opened any of his post. He merely collected it up, put it in a box, and when that box was full he sealed it and wrote the year on the top. When he died they found boxes and boxes of unopened post.

I've never taken the time to find out just how true this story is, but I do know that the first time I heard it, it had a profound effect on me and I wanted to do the same. However, being a somewhat deluded individual, I was fairly certain I could improve on the concept. Who, after all, would want to go through boxes of my unopened post?! Particularly when most of it would either be bills, red bills, final demands or letters from the utility companies informing me that I'd been cut off. I wanted my boxes to be full of interesting stuff.

And so I started to collect things. Ticket stubs mainly. Be they cinema or theatre tickets, raffle tickets, train tickets, plane tickets, pay-and-display parking tickets. But also postcards, greeting cards, thank you cards, business cards, labels, badges, old credit cards, menus, anything that was evidence of somewhere I'd been, something I'd done, or someone I'd seen or met.

I can't remember what I did with all this junk to start with, but eventually (probably in an effort to retain some sort of control over the growing mountain of rubbish) I decided to get a really large cork noticeboard and pin this stuff to it. And there it hung in my living room – a huge messy board packed with memories. I loved it!

A few months later, on New Year's Day, I completed the last stage of my 'Andy Warhol' project by removing everything from the board, stuffing it in the largest envelope I could find, writing the year on the front in huge letters, and tossing it in the loft. A few days later I started the process again, pinning items to the board as I accumulated them.

Now, many, many years later, I have approximately twenty huge envelopes in the loft, each one with a year written on the front, and each one packed with papery mementoes. Do I ever look in these envelopes? No. Will I? No. What's the point then?

The point isn't the envelopes. The point is the board. On the following page I present to the reader exhibit A:

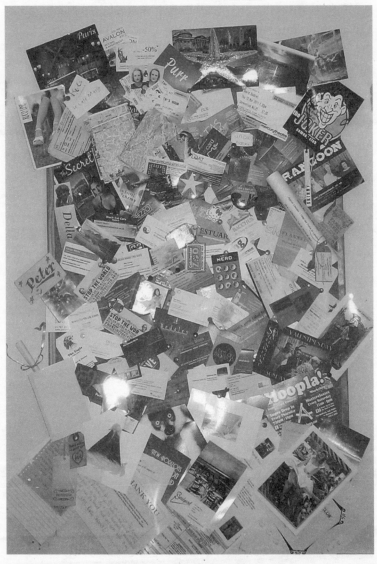

EXHIBIT A: MY TROPHY BOARD

That's 2011's board just before it was taken off the wall and all the items were tucked away in an envelope ready for the board to be repopulated throughout 2012. If you'd like to check my progress, visit the Facebook page,[17] or the blog.[18]

Some might say this is clutter. I've heard self-help gurus tell people that this sort of stuff has no place in your life. But to me the board is my 'Trophy Cabinet'. It's a visual reminder of all the things I've done this year, and the space between the items is an opportunity to be filled with something else. When visitors come round they stand and admire the board. It's a conversation piece. Sometimes people ask me to explain an item. Nobody ever tells me it's a bad idea.

And when I'm tired, or feeling low, or I'm feeling a little like a hamster on a wheel, and that nothing I do ever amounts to anything, I look at the board and I realise that it's not true. Twenty fat envelopes in my loft say otherwise.

17 www.facebook.com/howtodoeverythingandbehappy.com
18 www.howtodoeverythingandbehappy.com

STOP! ACTION POINT!

How to Create a Trophy Board

Take a BIG cork board ('A1' (approx 23×33 inches) is just about right). Find somewhere to hang it. Then start pinning tickets, photos, postcards … anything that'll remind you of moments that you've enjoyed during the year.

What you put on the board doesn't have to relate to your Now List. The idea here is to create a visual reminder of how fun your life is. Don't be put off by its initial emptiness, it'll fill up faster than you think – see the emptiness as an opportunity waiting to happen.

At the end of the year (or when the board's full – whatever works for you), take the items off, and if you want to, bag them up, label the bag, throw it in the loft. When your ceiling gives way under the weight and you're showered in plaster and papery items, you'll smile, knowing how fulfilling your life has been.

Taking the Trophy Board One Step Further

I love the messiness of the board. I love its randomness. I love how friends stand in front of it and see if they can find anything new. But I understand that there are those amongst you (with Virgo tendencies) who wouldn't be able to see past the scraps of paper. For you it would always be clutter – a mess – hanging on the wall.

So consider this. It doesn't have to be a board. Here are some other ideas I've experimented with.

Photos

When I was a kid cameras needed to be loaded with film. You could only take 36 pictures before the film was full and had to be developed – which cost money. Needless to say, as every single photo was being paid for out of my paper round money I thought very carefully about every image I took.

These days, however, photography is cheap. It's rare for me to go anywhere without a digital camera of some description. If I haven't got my trusty little compact Canon, my phone can do a fairly decent job at snapping the odd memory.

And I'm not the only one. My dear old Dad is the only member of my family who isn't packing a camera somewhere about his person whenever the family get together. Even my nephew and niece (who are six) have digital cameras.

Now more than ever aspects of my life are photographed from every angle several times a week, and not just by me, but also by friends and family.

So here's what I did recently. I spent a pleasant afternoon looking through pictures and every time I found one that made me smile I copied it into a different folder. Then I found one of those online photo printing companies (photobox.co.uk is pretty amazing), uploaded the photos to them, and I had them produce 6x4 prints. It cost me next to nothing – literally only pence per print – to have about fifty images printed on glossy photographic paper and mailed to me. The quality was outstanding, far better than I could have ever achieved myself.

My absolute favourites got pinned to the fridge, or on the wall in my office. The remainder I filed. Periodically I rearrange the photos, or replace them with fresh ones. At some point I'll print up some new ones.

For the clutter-phobic amongst you, you could consider investing in a digital photo frame. They're like laptop monitors without the keyboard attached. You simply insert a memory card into the back and the frame should cycle through your images like a screensaver on your computer.

At the time of writing these things vary in price and quality and I've discovered – to my cost – that there isn't necessarily a correlation between the two. However, if you manage to get a good one they're worth their weight in gold.

My advice is to avoid photo frames with built in speakers or rubbish that you don't need. You want the best screen quality you can get, at the cheapest price. Everything else is a bonus.

Scrap Books and Photo Books
Reader David dropped me a line:

'It occurred to me that you could stick the trophies from your trophy board into a scrap book, or scan them (the scannable ones anyway) and produce a 'photo book'.[19] That way, they don't get hidden away in the attic but can be a source of further inspiration for your next year.'

Great suggestion, David. I'm kicking myself for not thinking of it first.

Social Media

There's scientific evidence to suggest that telling someone about an experience you enjoyed reinforces that experience, and makes the happiness you derived from it last even longer.

Now obviously you could just phone up your friends and family and tell them all about it, but this is the digital age, and the one thing that technology has allowed us to do very effectively is to broadcast our innermost thoughts to the entire planet if we so desire. Even if you're a social media sceptic/cynic (and God knows I used to be) I encourage you to give the likes of Facebook and/or blogging a look. Used sensibly, they can be quite good fun.

Jars (and Similar)

Not all mementoes can be pinned to a notice board, fridge or uploaded to the internet. Every now and then you'll pick up something altogether more three-dimensional. Maybe a pebble from the beach. A pocket full of Lipa (Croatian

---

19 Companies such as photobox.co.uk and snapfish.co.uk give you the ability to produce some really stunning books from your own photos. Other companies offer similar services.

pennies). A finger puppet your niece made for you. A cork
from a bottle of champagne. The security pass from the time
you did a telly interview.

Don't throw these items into a drawer. Instead get
yourself an old-fashioned glass storage jar and start filling it
with this kind of stuff.

I like my jar because it's see-through. For me that adds
to its appeal. But your jar doesn't have to be a jar. My friend
Wendy has a 'memories trunk'. As do all her kids. My friend
Lynn has an old shoe box.

Not blowing your skirt up? Ok. I can respect that. Try this
for size:

Printer's Tray
Back in the old days (I'm talking really old – older than me –
long before computers, one might even say 'back in ancient
times'), newspapers were printed by taking small blocks of
metal, each of which had a letter embossed in the bottom, and
laying these blocks side by side in a tray to form words and
sentences. The blocks were wedged together, inked, and the
paper was quite literally 'stamped'.

As you can imagine, setting type was a time-consuming
business. To speed things up it was essential that these little
metal blocks were organised. And so they were. They were
kept in specially made drawers – trays – which themselves
were divided into sections.

What happened to these trays once the world went
computerised? Well, most were cast to one side. Some were
probably chopped up to make firewood. Others are probably
on a landfill site somewhere. A few, however, ended up being

sold at car boot or garage sales, and antique markets, and on eBay. I've just done a search and found 193 on sale, for about a tenner each.

And why should you care?

Printer's trays are absolutely perfect for all those little nick-nacks I mentioned above. Get yourself a tray, clean it up with wire wool, then screw it to the wall, and pretty soon you'll have something like the one on the following page.

Unlike the photos and the Trophy Board, the items in the printer's tray tend to stay in the same place year after year with only the occasional purge or addition. But that's just me. I can't even remember the significance of some of the items in the tray, but in a way I kinda like that. Like there's a memory there that's locked away and could only be retrieved by a particularly gifted hypnotist or psychic.

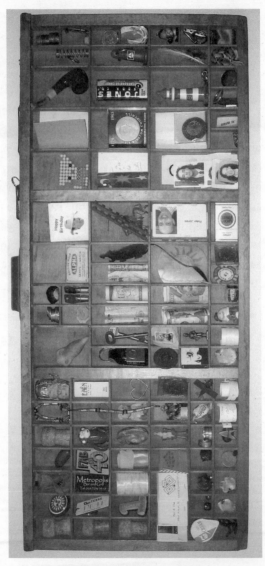

EXHIBIT B: MY PRINTER'S TRAY

Potential Now List Problems

Back to your Now List (which was how we got onto Trophy
Boards and the like). The rather wonderful thing about Now
Lists is that it seems there's very little that can go wrong! So
far there's only a handful of *challenges* that I've identified.

Money
If your Now List is anything like mine, there probably isn't
an item on the list that doesn't involve parting with money.
Which is annoying if you're strapped for cash, or on a
particularly tight budget.

Now you might be tempted to avoid adding items to
your list if they seem financially out of reach, but that would
be a mistake – any kind of censorship will only stifle your
creativity. Instead, create a Now List category called 'when I
have enough money' and add them anyway.

You might also want to consider starting a 'Now List
Fund'.

How you do that is entirely up to you. If you're like
me, setting up a 'fund' might only involve adding a line to
a spreadsheet somewhere, but if you're a normal person, or
someone who struggles to manage their finances, it might be
better to open a savings account, and maybe even one that
doesn't give you a cash card or internet banking or any other
easy way to access your money. You'll want to put your Now
List Fund out of easy reach.

You might also need to find creative ways of topping it up.

Jules (my long-suffering assistant) has a standing order set up to automatically put a small amount into her dedicated savings account each month. Even if you can only afford one pound/dollar/euro/drachma per month, it's one pound/dollar/euro/drachma in the right direction.

Personally I top up my Now List Fund whenever I'm given 'unexpected' money (e.g. if I win a tenner on the lottery or a premium bond pays out). But I also make my Now List available on the blog and on BucketList.org[20] and as a consequence family and friends often consult the list when looking for Birthday or Christmas gift ideas.

I appreciate however that money worries are crippling. If your financial situation is so dire that you can't, in good conscience, put aside any money to treat yourself, then bear with me a page or two longer. The next section is definitely for you.

What's the Difference between a Now List and a Potential Boxing Day List?

You might find, when compiling your Now List, or your Potential Boxing Day List, that you want to put the same item on both. Is that allowed?

The answer is yes, *so long as* the items on your Boxing Day List require no advance planning whatsoever (because that would break one of the rules of Boxing Day).

Personally I like the fact that I have two lists – one for items that require some planning and forethought, and one for

---

20   Other similar sites are available.

items that don't. But that's just me – if you want to duplicate items, knock yourself out.

'My [insert Now List activity] Was a Complete Failure!'
I'm sorry to hear that. What happened? Really? How awful. Allow me to share with you a similar story.

Shortly after launching the website to go along with this book I decided to start blogging about some of the items that I'd added to my Now List and succeeded in ticking off. One such item was this:

TRY A FLOTATION TANK EXPERIENCE

A 'flotation tank' (for those of you who are new to the concept) is a large bath filled with warm salt water and a sound proofed lid. Once the lid's closed the lights go off, leaving you floating in the dark, and the silence. The fact that most of your senses are deprived (you can't see anything, hear anything etc) allegedly allows your mind to enter a deeply relaxed state. One hour in the tank, so they say, is akin to several hours of fabulous relaxing sleep.

Unfortunately, on the day that I tried it I had a small paper cut on my thumb. Man – you do not want to get salt water on a paper cut! Neither do you want to thrash about in an effort to keep your thumb out of the water. You might end up splashing salt water on your face. Man – you do not want to get salt water into your eyes either!

Those thirty minutes in the tank (I got out early) felt like several hours of torture. If I'd had any secrets to tell I'd have spilled them after the first few minutes.

Not to be deterred, and determined to have something good to write for the blog, I booked a second flotation experience. This time I took up the offer of some optional 'relaxing' music. You know the sort of thing – pan pipes played softly against a background of waves bubbling over rock pools.

Unfortunately there was a problem with the CD player. Instead of drifting into the best sleep I've ever known, I lay in the dark, floating to a series of irritating clicks and buzzes.

I lasted fifteen minutes.

Finally, determined to make sure I got the best 'experience' possible, the flotation centre gave me a third, complimentary session, booked me into the most spacious state-of-the-art pod they had, and double checked everything.

I lay there for fifty minutes.

Nothing hurt.

There was no buzzing.

But my God, I was so bored.

I did have plenty of time to think, though, and as I gently tapped the side of the pod and floated from one side to the other I began to realise that actually, flotation might be overrated. My own bath is pretty darn nice. It sits under a huge window. And if you open that window on a summer's day there's really nothing better than lying up to your chin in soapy bath water – that won't irritate your paper cuts – whilst looking up at the puffy white clouds, and listening to the sound of the birds chirping and generally being terrorised by my cat.

I got out of the tank, went home, and did exactly that.

Was my flotation tank experience a wash-out?

Yes. Yes it was.

But does that mean that my *next* Now List activity will be a disaster?

Of course not.

But then I'm sure you realised that.

Feeling Happier?

So how are you? How are you feeling? How's your Now List looking? Got anything planned? Checked any items off yet? And whilst I'm firing off questions, when was your last Boxing Day? Really? Maybe you should have another one soon, eh?

If this all feels like 'frosting', as Americans would call it – if it feels a bit like we're filling our days with sugary treats but no real substance, or covering over our fundamentally sad existence with a layer of sickly sweet icing – then I would respectfully ask you to stick with me just a little while longer. In the next section we're going to break through the icing and the marzipan, and move into the cake.

We're going to tackle the big stuff.

We're going to find out what it is that you actually want.

Pointing Your Life in a Better Direction

What Do You Want?

What is it that you want? Right now?

Maybe you want a nice cup of tea, the people next door to turn down their music, and an end to war, poverty and Mariah Carey cover versions? These are all good.

But what about your life?

What would make it better?

What would make you happier?

What do you want?

Most people I encounter haven't actually got a clue what they really want. They might wake up in the morning and *want* to go back to bed. They might flick through a magazine and *want* those shoes. They might even *want* the person, in the magazine, wearing those shoes. But these desires come and go. Few of them seem to stick around and become important – which is odd because when you're growing up, figuring out *what you want* is very important and actively encouraged.

'What do you want for Christmas?'

'What do you want to do today?'

'What do you want to be when you grow up?'

A huge part of being a kid is spent working out what we want, and then writing it down or telling someone about it. And yet, as we get older, and we're finally in a position to do something about the bigger 'wants' of our childhood, we seem to give the question less and less thought. As if the day-to-day grind of making ends meet is more than enough to occupy every waking minute.

And that's a mistake.

Knowing exactly what you want is hugely important. Merely *knowing* has the power to change *everything*.

Not convinced? Then allow me to introduce you to the incredible, completely automated wish-fulfilment machine you have inside your head.

The Power of Focus

Brains are amazing. Especially yours. Even mine has its moments. And one of the most fascinating mechanisms of the human brain is how it deals with 'focus'.

Have you ever noticed how when you buy a new car, or even when you've merely decided what type of car it is you want to buy, you start seeing that same car everywhere?!

Or the kettle packs up, the DVD stops playing, and suddenly half a dozen other electrical items in the house decide to turn up their boots, like they're all suffering from some sort of appliance manic depression.

Or how you can sleep through a thunderstorm, the traffic noise, and the sounds of revellers returning from a night on the town, but if your newborn's breathing changes even slightly – *in the next room* – you're awake!

Or have you ever seen someone across a crowded room, started to walk towards them, and somehow walked into the table, the person, the immovable object, that was directly in front of you but momentarily invisible?

Or have you ever fallen in love, fallen out of love, had a tiff, a blazing row, a passing thought about that girl you used to know – and the words of the next song on the radio seem to capture your feelings precisely?

That's the power of focus. And it happens because in order for our brains to cope with the extraordinary amount of information coming in through our five senses from the world around us, we're programmed to concentrate on what's 'important' and more or less ignore the rest.

Unconvinced? Excellent!

Pick a card from the six on the opposite page. Don't tell me which one it is, just pick one, and remember which card you've chosen.

No, don't pick the King of Spades, everyone picks that one! Pick a different card.

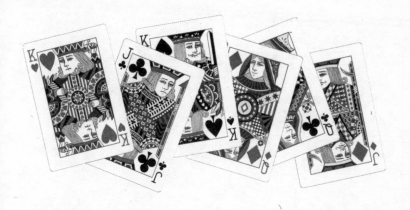

Ready?
Now turn the page.

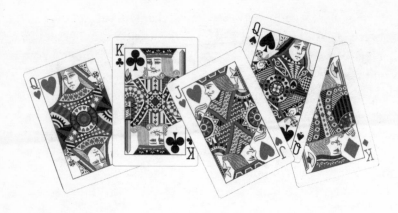

And it's gone!

But curiously enough, so has the King of Spades, and yet there are still five cards left. How is that possible?

Before you start flipping backwards and forwards between pages to figure out how I did that (if you haven't figured it out already), have you got access to the internet? If so, log onto www.howtodoeverythingandbehappy.com/focus and watch the short Selective Attention video. When you're done, you can come back here and turn the page.

WARNING: TURNING THE PAGE
BEFORE WATCHING THE VIDEO
WILL RENDER THE EXPERIMENT USELESS

So, what's going on in your head that you can watch a short video of kids playing basketball and utterly fail to notice something so obvious? The answer, of course, is 'focus'. Your mind was concentrating on something else, just as in the card trick you were concentrating on the card you'd chosen, and its apparent disappearance, and failed entirely to notice that all the cards had changed. The other cards weren't 'important'.

You might be asking yourself how does the brain determine what's important? And the answer is: you tell it! In both of the experiments it was you who chose what to focus on.

And this mechanism isn't just taking place during card tricks and basketball games; this happens all day, every day. Your brain is continually filtering the information coming in, based on what you've decided is important.

Strange then that we quite often focus on entirely the wrong things, or nothing at all.

Focusing on the Wrong Things

It's a curious thing, but in driving incidents where a motorist loses control of their vehicle (say, in icy conditions) it's surprising how often they manage to hit a solitary tree, lamp post, or other static object, when statistically they should have been far more likely to have come to a halt on the other side of the road, or in a field.

This is because in those crucial seconds when they're spinning out of control your average driver will concentrate on trying *not* to hit the tree or the lamp post. Put another way, their focus will be on the very thing they don't want to hit, and as a consequence – they hit it!

This might seem crackers to you – it did to me. Were I to skid off the road I too would be gripping the steering wheel, looking at that tree, and doing everything in my power to avoid it. But as any racing driver might tell you, what I should be looking at is *where I want to be,* i.e. the road.

The same thing apparently applies to showjumpers. They're taught to look beyond the jump – where they need to be. Look at the hedge and the horse will often stop abruptly, catapulting the rider into the air, with only the hard ground or brambles to break their fall.

This isn't just a top driving or showjumping tip; this goes for life in general. What you should focus on is where you want to be.

It might sound obvious, it might even be what you *think* you're doing, but have you ever started a sentence with the words 'I don't want …' or 'If only I wasn't …' or 'There has to be something better than …'? If so, you are focusing on what you DON'T want, and consequently you're subconsciously steering your life in the wrong direction. It's how the brain works. It's almost as if the brain can't process the 'negative' element. 'Don't hit that tree' becomes 'hit that tree'.

Did I hear someone make a comment about manure? Not convinced, eh? Ok. Try this simple experiment. Ready?

DO NOT THINK ABOUT A BOX OF FROGS.

I'll bet my book royalties that by the time you made it to the end of the sentence there was a box of frogs sitting slap bang in the middle of your imagination.

It simply isn't possible to *not* focus on something. The very act of NOT thinking about something requires your brain to conjure up images of the thing you don't want to think about, so you can ignore it.

The only way to avoid focusing on the wrong thing is to switch your focus to something else. Which, it has to be said, is far easier said than done. Particularly if you've made focusing on the wrong things a habit.

A couple of years ago I went away for a few days with a friend who really struggles to focus on the positive. One afternoon, as we sat outside a bar, drinking cold beers in the blazing heat, my friend – who had somehow failed to enjoy two days of glorious sunshine, fantastic food, and bustling streets – turned to me and said, 'So, what would you say has been your biggest disappointment of this holiday?'

It wasn't a question I wanted to answer. Yes, there were things that I could have thought of – if I'd tried – but the question revolted me. I didn't want to start making a list of *disappointments*; for one thing, my travelling companion would have been at the top of the list! But more than that, it would have meant focusing on the wrong things. It would have been telling my brain to be on the lookout for 'disappointments', to expect a negative outcome – just as my companion had – and pretty soon I'd have been sitting there feeling just as miserable.

Your brain is amazing. It'll take you in whatever direction you tell it. And if, like my friend, you've got into the habit of telling it to fill your days with disappointment, failure, worry and sadness it'll definitely deliver.

However, you can use that *same* mental process to turn your life around by focusing on an outcome you actually want – my wife used to say, 'Worry about things going well.'

Continuously focus your brain on the outcome you want and you'll find yourself achieving goals, experiencing success and feeling happier.

Focusing on Nothing

Allow me to tell you another tale.

It had been twenty years since we'd last seen each other.

A lot can happen in twenty days, even twenty minutes can be quite eventful, so it was probably unreasonable to expect to cover the events of twenty years in the time it took to drink a mug of hot chocolate. It was, however, just enough time to get the general gist, and the gist was this: in those twenty years things hadn't worked out so well for my friend. She was very, very unhappy.

Life hadn't been a disaster – not in the slightest – but it certainly wasn't where she hoped it would be. She had a part-time job she didn't really enjoy. She was married to a man she wasn't in love with. And they lived in a house that was far too small, in a rough little neighbourhood, miles from anyone.

I couldn't understand it. When we were at school this girl had everything going for her – she was smart, funny, gorgeous – somehow it just didn't make sense that her life wasn't more … well, more!

And so we met for coffee again. And again. And again. And each week she'd tell me how this year's holiday would once again be spent in a caravan in Bognor. Not that there's anything wrong with Bognor, but after fifteen years it was beginning to lose its sparkle.

Or how, just for once, it would be nice to watch TV without having to move the computer desk first.

Or how every time she climbed into a bubble bath for a long soak, one of the kids, even her husband, always needed to use the toilet. If only they had a downstairs loo...

The list went on.

And on.

After the third week my sympathy was beginning to wane. It wasn't that my friend was complaining about nothing – her gripes were, in many ways, justified. And if her situation had been brought about by a spell of rotten luck – something outside of her control – I'd have gushed sympathy till it came out of my ears, but from what I could see every single unsatisfactory element of her life had been the consequence of a decision that she had, at some point, been involved in.

For instance, fifteen years of Bognor holidays was something she'd elected to do – she and her husband. True, her husband is a man who's a little stuck in his ways. True, their budget was quite limited. But it was hard to believe that a caravan in Bognor was the *only* family holiday option available, for fifteen years running.

Likewise the tiny house. At some point a decision had been made to buy that house, in that area. Again, finances had been an issue, *but there would have been options*. Surely? But from what I could discern, my friend had actually let her husband find and pick the house.

And let's talk about him – the husband. You might be wondering if she'd married a man who *changed*, or turned out to have a wicked streak. That can happen. Happens all the time. But from what I could tell she never really liked him. Ever. But she'd married him anyway. In fact, it would be more accurate to say he'd married her, and she'd merely turned up at the church at the allotted time.

It was thoughts like these that would float around my head as I sipped my hot chocolate and listened to another episode of 'woe is me'. And as our coffee meet-ups appeared to be getting longer and longer, I had more and more time to dwell on my friend's predicament. Until one day she said:

'I like our coffee meet-ups. I get so bored during the day.'

'Bored?' I replied.

'God, yes.' I bit my lip. Boredom is a concept I have strong feelings about.

'So what does your typical day involve?' I asked.

'Well, obviously I have to get the kids up,' she said.

'Of course,' I said.

'And make their sandwiches.'

'Very important.'

'And make sure they have everything they need – PE kits, books …'

'Sure,' I said.

'Then I have to take them to school.'

'Right.'

'Then I might have to take them to their after-school clubs.'

'Uh huh.'

'Help them with their homework.'

'Mmm.'

'Then I cook dinner, tidy up, get things ready for the morning, then we're into our bedtime routine—'

'Ok, ok – what about whilst they're at school?'

'Well, Tuesday and Thursday I work in the shop …'

'Yes.'

'Wednesday I see you.'

'For an hour.'

'Or two,' she said with a smile.

'Ok. And the rest of the time?' She thought for a moment. Thought really hard. I was expecting her to tell me how much work it was to keep the house tidy, or maybe she went shopping, or visited her mother.

'Well, I guess I might watch a bit of telly. Maybe read a magazine?' And there it was. That told me everything I needed to know. The real answer to what my friend did with her time, aside from all the things she *had* to do, in the morning, and the evenings, was *precisely nothing*.

In fact 'precisely nothing' was the effort she'd put in to taking charge of her life from the very moment she left school. Her holidays, her house, even her husband was a direct result of absolutely zero effort on her part.

Put like that, her life didn't seem so bad – in fact, her life was an absolutely fabulous return on her zero investment.

It's easy for me to sound righteous here, but in fact there are many, many examples I could use from my own life where, due to a total lack of effort, *lack of focus*, on my part, I ended up with a situation that was less than satisfactory. I call it Living by Default.

Living by Default appears to happen whenever we assume that things will work out ok because *they should*, and/ or we've expended very little effort on deciding what it is in life we actually want.

For instance, when I was a much younger man I naturally assumed that I would meet someone, fall in love, get married and have kids. I wasn't particularly fussy about who that someone might be, how or when this great romance was going to happen, or anything about the kids other than there would probably be some. I was just happy to wait and let it happen. That was, after all, how life was supposed to work.

It was only in my thirties, when I noticed that people had stopped describing me as an 'eligible bachelor' and started instead to question my sexuality, that I realised that there was quite a strong chance that the woman of my dreams was not going to knock on the door and invite herself into my life. Believe me when I tell you this was a shock. Due to my complete and total lack of focus on the relationship front, Life had delivered to me my default setting – i.e. no one.

My friend and fellow author Wendy Steele says, 'A life lived in fear is a life half lived.' I'd like to suggest that Living by Default has the potential to be worse. You only have one life. And if you choose to let it take you where it wants, like a leaf floating in a stream with dreams of someday reaching the ocean, that's your decision to make – just don't complain to me if you find yourself trapped on the rocks, or snagged by overhanging branches.

If, on the other hand, you'd rather not leave your happiness to chance, well that's an altogether more exciting attitude and something I'd very much like to be a part of.

What are you waiting for? Let's get started.

And where do we start?

By figuring out what it is you actually want.

Making a Wish List

Imagine that, in a moment of madness, you've decided to start redecorating. And I don't mean just slapping a fresh coat of paint on the walls – I mean major changes to your living space, the sort that involve a lump hammer being taken to that annoying dividing wall – and, in the process of undermining the structural integrity of your home, you discover an ancient-looking oil lamp within the wall cavity. You take off your rubber goggles, pick up the lamp, give it a rub and hey presto – an eight-foot genie is standing amongst the plaster and broken tiles.

'Master,' he says, 'I have the power to grant thee three wishes.' Three wishes? you think. That's handy.

So what would they be?

Now, don't just sit there staring into space whilst you ponder that. *This is important* and requires a little more than reeling off the first three things that come to mind. The genie isn't going anywhere – you have some time, so let's do this properly.

Grab a pen and a piece of paper and just start writing things down. Go ahead – you can do this now whilst you read this book. If you haven't got a pen or paper to hand (and it's too much effort to reach for the drawer that you keep your collection of cheap biros in) then create a 'note' on your mobile phone, or whatever gadget you have to hand. If you happen to be sitting in a café, squirt some ketchup on a napkin and use a breadstick like a quill pen. Whatever it takes. But you need to be able to jot down some thoughts, whatever comes into that mind of yours when faced with the question on the following page …

What do you want?

Don't over-think it – write down everything. And I mean *everything*. Because it turns out that whilst genies enforce a three wish limit, there's nothing to stop you coming back for a second or third round of wishes. It's a bandwidth issue. Not storage. You can, in fact, have as many wishes as you like, limited only by the bounds of your own lifetime. So go wild.

There are two important things you need to bear in mind.

IMPORTANT THING NUMBER 1:
YOU'LL BE DOING A LOT OF THE WORK
(OR, AT THE VERY LEAST, ORGANISING IT).

(Sorry about that. Previous stories about genies granting wishes with little or no effort on the part of the wisher were a slight exaggeration.)

IMPORTANT THING NUMBER 2:
ALL WISHES HAVE TO BE WITHIN
THE BOUNDS OF POSSIBILITY
AND PHYSICS.

So, for instance, whilst '*Become invisible so I can sneak into my local football stadium*' might seem like a fantastic wish, one that would significantly add to your quality of life, unless you're willing to put in a significant amount of effort into discovering how to bend light around yourself at will, it might be a whole lot quicker and easier to change your wish to '*Buy a season ticket*'.

You started writing yet? Come on. You can write and read. How about you write down three things before you continue?

Chunk Down

It's often useful to break your wishes into smaller sub-wishes, or to create a list of related wishes.

For instance, you might write:

Learn to play an instrument.

Then follow it up with:

Learn to play the guitar.

Then follow it up with:

Buy a guitar!

Then follow it up with:

Play in a band.

Then follow it up with:

Write a hit single and tour the world.

… and these things are all great. Let's try not to get stuck on one train of thought, though. Now that we've covered your musical ambition, let's move on to something else. What else would you like?

What do you want?

Sell Yourself Short. Or Long

Some people, when faced with a task like this, engage in some 'inner censorship'. They go to write down what they want – and then they stop themselves. And ninety-nine times out of a hundred it's because of fear.

Fear of ridicule from others.

Fear that their wishes might be impossible.

Fear of setting themselves up for some future failure.

Fear of acknowledging some inner voice that they've spent a lifetime ignoring.

Let me try and relieve you of that fear.

This is *just a list*. That's all. Just a piece of paper with thoughts on it. We're just writing things down. And – unless you have a burning desire to do otherwise – this is your Wish List *and should remain private*!

So, this being the case, it's fine to think big.

Want to walk on the moon? Write that down. Become President? Of the world? Write that down. Show Mariah Carey how to cover a record without butchering it? Definitely write that down.

It's also fine to think small.

So you really want those shoes? Fine! Shoes are important. Write that down! You want time to watch *EastEnders* each evening? I can't think of anything worse, but it's not *my* list – write it down. You want to read more often, get out in the garden once a week, work your way through all those Jamie Oliver cookbooks – then for heaven's sake, *write those things down*.

Stay in the Positive

It's a funny thing about working out what we want. It's often easier to think about what we *don't* want.

People will say things like:

'I don't want to work another day in this crappy dead-end job!'

Or: 'I don't want to come home to a pile of problems and things that need sorting out!'

Or: 'I don't want to go out with someone like him/her again!'

But none of these things are *'what you want'* – instead, as we discussed earlier in the chapter, they're focusing your mind on the very opposite.

But, you might be thinking, isn't figuring out what you DON'T want a good place to start?

For instance, if your crappy dead-end job is getting you down, then surely a better job – one where you're valued and appreciated, and there are prospects – would be something you *want*, right?

If you don't want to come home to a pile of problems, isn't it only reasonable to assume that you'd prefer to come home to ... something else? Maybe your spouse and your kids lined up, ready to greet you?

If the radio's playlist is getting you down then surely what you want is ... better tunes on the radio? A different radio station? A CD player? An iPod?

Not necessarily.

People fall into two distinct groups. Those that 'run away from' things, and those that 'run towards' things.

Most people, myself included, are in the first group. This isn't necessarily a bad thing. By and large, a 'running away from' strategy will work, and keep you safe, *in the short term*. If, for instance, you're out foraging for food and you happen to see a sabre-toothed tiger in the undergrowth, a 'running away from' strategy is a very good thing.

It's not so great when it comes to figuring out what you want from life, though. And (as in the examples above) merely working out the 'wants' from the 'don't wants' is still nothing more than a 'running away from' strategy in disguise.

Using a 'running away from' strategy to chart the course of your life is a little like embarking on a journey to some far flung destination merely by trying to get as far away from your current location as possible, and without knowing where you want to get to. It might work – possibly – but it's extremely unlikely. To stand any real chance of ending up in the right place you need to know exactly where you want to be and, if possible, a general direction.

It might help to make sure each sentence starts with the words 'I want' and beware of any sentences that contain negative words such as 'stop', 'not' or 'end'.

For instance, you might think you want to *quit* smoking. And there are many, many people in this world who have done exactly that. They quit smoking, and they're still *quitting*. They've been counting the minutes, days, sometimes years, since their last cigarette. It's as if at any moment they might crack under the pressure of not smoking, grab the nearest packet of Marlboros, light one up, and cough a huge sigh of relief.

I'd like to suggest that maybe what you *really* want is to 'be a non-smoker'. Non-smokers don't live their lives in the shadow of the last cigarette, they just live. Usually for longer. They don't even think of themselves as *non*-smokers, in the same way that I don't think of myself as a *non*-female. Non-smokers are just ... we're ... well, we're people who breathe clean, regular air rather than anything else. There. Clean air breathers. That's what's we are.

Have a quick look at what you've written so far. If you've got any negative wishes on your list, consider weeding them out and then asking yourself what it is that you *really* want.

Engage Your Inner Lawyer

Genies can be sneaky. If there's an easier way of granting your wish without actually achieving what you *really* meant that's exactly what will happen.

Let me give you an example.

You might say that you want to quit your boring office job.

No – you don't.

For one thing, that's a horrible negative wish, but much more seriously, for the Genie to grant that wish all he or she needs to do is arrange for you to be fired, or made redundant, leaving you without the boring office job and any form of income.

'Ok,' you might say, 'in that case, I want a better job.'

Better? Better how? What if the Genie arranged for you to receive a promotion; more money, more responsibility, more hours …

'No, no, no,' you say, 'I want to work somewhere else, for more money, less hours, and within an hour of my home.'

Excellent. In that case I have a vacancy that might interest you. You would be our Senior Clothing Research Technician with special responsibility for Mono-Chrome Fastening Devices for a small but select group of our customers. We need you to find and separate all the left-handed black and white buttons from this big pile in the corner.

To which you'd reply: 'I want to *enjoy* working somewhere else for more money, less hours, and within an hour of my home.'

Good for you. Now you're getting somewhere.

And You Want That Because?

So how many items have you got on your list so far?

Here's a little exercise for you. Run down the list and in your head ask yourself: 'Why do I want this?'

Take Beth, for instance. At the top of her Wish List she's written: 'I want to date George Clooney.'

And why do you want that, Beth?

Beth thinks long and hard about this (after I've dismissed her rather glib answer that George is 'fit' and what woman wouldn't want to be dating him!)

'Because I want a fit boyfriend,' says Beth. And just like that we've uncovered an underlying wish. She wants a boyfriend. A fit one. Let's see if we can go deeper still. Why do you want a boyfriend? What's the wish beneath this one?

'Because I don't want to be alone.'

That's a '*running away from*' strategy.

'Because I want to share my life with someone nice.'

Much better. And you want that because?

'That would make me happy.'

All your wishes should eventually get back to this point. If they don't, then I'd argue that they have no place on your Wish List. But think carefully before assuming that your desire for happiness is the layer beneath whatever wishes you have on your list – most wishes have several layers. This exercise can, when done carefully, uncover some very interesting, very personal desires that shed light on what it *really* is that would make you happy.

And that is, after all, the point of this book.

STOP! ACTION POINT!

Consider creating a Wish List

Ask yourself the question: 'What do you want?'

Keep in mind these important points:
1. You can have as many wishes as you want
2. Keep your wishes within the bounds of possibility and the laws of physics
3. Break your wishes into smaller and/or subsequent wishes
4. Think about all the different aspects of your life – don't get hung up on one thing
5. Feel free to think as big as you like
6. Or small. Be honest with yourself
7. Make all wishes positive – avoid 'running away from' strategies
8. Be absolutely clear on what you want. Leave the Genie no room to wriggle out. Engage your inner lawyer
9. Think about the wish beneath your wish – the layer below. Is there something more fundamental that should be on your list instead of, or as well as, the top layer?

The Power of Three

Hopefully what you have in front of you now is a page or two
(maybe more) of 'wishes'.

Now the work really begins.

Take a fresh sheet of paper (open a new document, create a
new note – whatever) and, referring back to your Wish List,
pick out the three 'wishes' – just three – that you would like
to achieve first. We'll come back to the others later, I promise,
but for now pick the three things from your list that you want
most in life.

So, for instance – getting back to your musical ambitions
– whilst all the things you wrote down were great (the world
tour sounds absolutely fab – please feel free to invite me to
the after show party), 'learn to play the guitar' is an obvious
first step on your road to fame and fortune, and would
therefore make a good first *wish*.

Try and make sure that the items you pick are achievable
in the next year or two. Whilst I don't have a problem with
long term wishes they have a nasty habit of staying long term.
So if your wish is 'world domination' – and you realise that
this might take four or five years to achieve – create a smaller
wish first: 'Purchase island in the South Pacific and build evil
mastermind lair' or 'Create robot army' springs to mind.

It's up to you, but I like to pick three wishes that reflect
three very different areas of my life. Say, my work life, my
personal life, and … something else.

You're probably wondering why I've limited you to three wishes. Why spend all that time creating a thirty-page Wish List if at the end of the day you're only going to work on three of them at once? Why not work on them all?!

The sad fact is there is only one of you. Only one person to get the work done. To have the absolute best chance of success, when it comes to turning your wishes into reality you need to limit how many you work on simultaneously.

Like everything in this book, I learned this lesson by bitter experience. Not so long ago my 'daily' to-do list ran to *sixteen pages of A4*. As you might expect of a man who's quite keen on organisation and planning, the list was basically every single thing I had to do for every project and goal I wanted to achieve. As a result my days quite often felt like I was nudging several hundred dominoes forward a centimetre at a time, and when I had nudged forward the last domino I would collapse into bed, weary and dejected, only to start again the following day.

Nothing in my life seemed to move forward very fast.

Then I listened to *Work Less, Make More*, by Jennifer White, and was intrigued by a principle called 'the power of three'. Concentrate on only three things at once, says Jennifer. Just three. Within each project focus only on the three tasks that will help you complete the project. If these tasks can be broken down further – into sub-steps – concentrate on only three of those steps. Everything else goes on the backburner.

'The power of three,' says Jennifer, 'will set you free.'

You can use 'the power of three' in almost everything, and it's especially powerful if you're the kind of person who finds it easy to start something, but difficult to finish.

Implement this principle and you simply won't be able to start something new until at least one of your existing three 'projects' is complete.

For instance, if you've bought a wreck of a house and you plan to renovate the whole thing, the power of three would dictate that you pick only three rooms to start with – maybe the kitchen, the bathroom and a bedroom. Within those three rooms you'll pick a maximum of three tasks to start and complete; so within the bathroom you might decide to rip out the existing suite, chip off the old tiles and replace the windows – but you won't start pulling up the floorboards and messing with the pipes until one of the other items is complete.

My house decorating analogy might not work in reality – DIY is not my strong suit. However, I implemented the power of three into my mammoth to-do list and suddenly my life started moving forwards. As of today the to-do list is only six pages long (I just checked).

But I digress. Back to wishes … Time for you to do some work.

STOP! ACTION POINT!

Pick three wishes from your Wish List

- Pick the three that are the most important to you
- *Consider* picking three wishes from different 'areas' of your life

Use the Power of Focus

Remember we talked about your brain's extraordinary ability to focus? Of course you do. It was only a few pages ago. This being the case – and you being the wonderfully astute person that you are – you're probably wondering if we can use this power of focus to make all those things on your Wish List come true.

The answer is yes – yes we can.

There are numerous techniques I use, the most powerful of which is to take your three wishes and turn them into 'goals'. We'll look at this in the next section; for now, however, I want to reiterate that *simply knowing* what it is that you want has already started to re-programme your subconscious. You'll be surprised at how this affects what you notice, or don't notice, over the next few days.

But just to be sure, here are two or three easy suggestions to help get those wishes into your head and reinforce your power of focus.

Review Your Three Wishes Every Day
How you do this is up to you, but see if you can create a habit whereby you remind yourself of your top three wishes. Good times to do this might be …

- As you brush your teeth (shower, blow-dry your hair)
- As you drive to work (walk to the station, drive the kids to school)
- As you walk up the stairs (a different wish for each flight of steps, maybe)

The Wish Board / Screensaver / Mug

Remember the Trophy Board we created in the Now List section? The board covered with ticket stubs, photos, and all manner of Now List memorabilia? It's worth creating a second board – *a Wish Board* – stuffed with imagery of what you'd like in your life. For many years my wife and I had a board like this in our kitchen.

A Wish Board like this works in two ways – not only is the board itself a visual reminder of your wishes, but the act of keeping an eye out for appropriate images as you leaf through magazines is in itself an exercise in programming your subconscious.

If you don't subscribe to any magazines, sit down at your computer, bring up Google, and perform an 'image search'. You can print those images out for your board and/or save those images[21] into a 'folder' on your computer and use the slideshow screensaver (almost every computer has one) to display these pictures whenever the computer's idle.

---

21 To save a picture from a webpage, <u>right</u> click the image – you'll usually be offered the option to save the image on your computer.

STOP! ACTION POINT!

Harness your power of focus!

Knowing what you want momentarily points your subconscious in the right direction. Reminding yourself creates more of those moments.
- Run through your three wishes daily
- Consider creating a Wish Board
- Create a Wish Screensaver

Potential Wish List Problems

Right now, I estimate there's an 80% chance that you'll be basking in the clarity of having worked out exactly what it is that you want out of life. Over the coming days your family and friends will pick up magazines only to notice that some of the pages are missing, where you've torn out an inspirational image. People will catch you sitting in front of your computer watching the screensaver, or talking to yourself in front of the bathroom mirror. And you'll start to notice 'stuff'.

For instance, maybe you've already noticed that there's a car, pretty much identical to the one you've always wanted, sitting in the showroom of that second-hand car dealership just down the road. Or the local college is running an evening class in South American basket weaving, a skill you've always wanted to develop – what were the chances? Or last night you happened to overhear a guy in the pub telling someone how he's planning on starting a petition to ask Mariah Carey to cease from making any more cover versions. This is the power of focus at work. Your subconscious is busy identifying things that you've deemed important to you, and putting them on the radar of your mind, in case you want to do something about it.

Now, whilst 80% is a fairly good percentage, I can't really continue without trying to address the 20% of people who are sitting there with a bewildered, grumpy or downright frustrated expression. Let's go over some common Wish List problems.

I'm Confused! What's the Difference between My Wish List and My Now List?

You might find that having diligently written your Now List in the previous section, you now want to write exactly the same things on your Wish List. Is that ok?

Possibly.

Your Now List is the answer to this question:

WHAT WOULD I LIKE TO EXPERIENCE
BEFORE I DIE?

Your Wish List is the answer to this question:

WHAT DO I WANT
[IN MY LIFE] OR [MY LIFE TO BE]?

Now it may be that, when faced with either question, you immediately think 'climb Mount Kilimanjaro'! And that's just fine. Clearly climbing this mountain is an experience – therefore making your Now List – and you obviously feel so strongly about it that when faced with a genie this would be your first wish – thereby making your Wish List.

In practice, however, it doesn't *really* matter. If, by putting an item on your Now List and/or your Wish List, it ends up being something that you do, and that makes you happy – then good for you. My work here is done.

I've got more to say on this subject, but I'd like to come back to it at the end of the next section if that's ok with you.

It's All Me, Me, Me, Me, Me!

It's no fun growing up with brothers and sisters. Life is a constant battle for supremacy. And whilst being the eldest, or the tallest, or the strongest, should give you the competitive edge amongst your siblings, there's always a parent hovering in the background who's just one squabble away from wading in and levelling the playing field with a clip round the ear and comments such as:

'Wait your turn,' or

'Be nice to your sister,' or

'How many times have I told you to share?!'

You can appeal, of course – I often did – but this was usually met with:

'Peter – not everything's about you,' or

'If you can't play nicely then I'll take it away,' or

'I want, I want, I want – that's all I ever hear!'

It seems that no sooner have we been encouraged to 'think for ourselves' and 'decide what we want in life' than someone, maybe the same someone, tells us that we're being self-centred or selfish. 'Putting others first,' so they say, is the true path to enlightenment.

Now I'm not going to tell you that our parents were wrong – not entirely – but a few of us (and I include myself in this) had this concept of putting others first beaten into us so effectively that we've all but lost the ability to consider our own needs, and to do so can often fill us with feelings of guilt. That's not good.

What our parents should have told us was this:

TAKING INTO CONSIDERATION OUR OWN WANTS

TO THE EXCLUSION OF EVERYONE ELSE

IS WRONG.

The middle line of that sentence is crucial! Without it, you're effectively telling yourself that everyone else is more important than you – and whilst there will be those of you who actually believe that, <u>it's simply not true</u>.

Here's another thing your parents should have told you:

TAKING INTO CONSIDERATION EVERYONE ELSE

TO THE EXCLUSION OF YOURSELF

IS UTTERLY, UTTERLY WRONG.

No good can come of thinking of others to the exclusion of yourself. You will end up standing in the Personal Growth aisle of your local bookshop, real or virtual, considering books on how to become happier.

However, these can be *incredibly hard* concepts to grasp. From the workshops I run I've found that mums especially are often hard-wired to put their own needs or wants on the back burner, or to dismiss them completely. So even if you finally manage to get your logical brain to say, 'Oh yes, I see now – I need to strike a balance,' your inner child will continue to follow the put-everyone-else-first rule in the hope that one day it'll magically start working for you.

It won't.

And sadly, undoing this level of brainwashing takes more than a couple of pages in a book like this.

All that said, there are a few things you could try.

Firstly, there's therapy. And I'm not kidding. It really is the only way to free yourself from this noble, but nonetheless destructive, behaviour. A word of warning: therapy is like embarking on a long personal journey through your own psyche for which you really need a qualified and experienced guide. Finding a therapist that works for you can be a challenge. This isn't a reason not to try therapy; just try, if you can, to see a therapist who someone you trust can recommend.

Secondly, you could leave yourself notes around your house or office to remind you of the two facts above. Will it work? Maybe. It's a low-tech solution that won't remedy the underlying problem, but sometimes a quick fix is all that's necessary to enable us to continue on in life.

Lastly, you could strike a compromise with yourself. Accept the fact that there are other people in your life and incorporate them into your Wish List. Grab a piece of paper and instead of starting your wishes with the words 'I want', try starting a few with 'we want' and see where that gets you.

For instance:

'We want to travel the world.'

'My mother and I live in a wonderful house, near the sea.'

'I am learning to play the guitar, with the support of …'

Knowing What You Really Want Is Hard!

Lucy says:

'I find it utterly laudable in intention that you're inviting people to identify what they truly want and take responsibility for getting it – but I am brought up short by the fact that you make no reference to how HARD it is to find out what we *really truly want, as opposed to what we are culturally invited to find desirable.'*

You're right. It is hard to find out what you really truly want. Perhaps it even borders on the impossible. So my advice to you is to STOP trying to find out what you *'really truly want'* and instead answer the infinitely simpler question:

What do you want?

Don't over-think it. Don't edit yourself. Don't dismiss the first thought that comes to mind. This is a book on becoming happy, not spiritually fulfilled. If you want to *eat chocolate every single day*, write that down. If you want to *lose weight from a lifetime of eating chocolate every day,* write that down. Just ask yourself the question – then write! If you haven't got an answer by the end of this paragraph chances are you're thinking way too deep! You'll find the very act of creating a Wish List sparks off new ideas – and who knows, eventually one of them might be the Holy Grail that you're looking for, the thing you *really truly want.*

In the meantime, shift your focus away from 'how difficult it is' and get writing.

The 'Universe' and Its Wicked Sense of Humour
It's a funny thing about the focus mechanism in your head. As well as bringing to your attention all those things you've deemed important, you may find you start to notice all the things that are, on the face of it, the complete opposite.

Say, for instance, that your three wishes basically amount to the same thing: 'Spend more time with the family.' You've created yourself a nice screensaver featuring pictures of you and the kids, and the walls of your office are now plastered with family photos. No sooner have you done this than your boss walks in and offers you a raise. And a promotion. And a new car. And an expense account. And a bigger office. In Dubai. For six months.

Now clearly this job in Dubai runs counter to your wish. It is, nonetheless, a very exciting opportunity. You might even do a little detective work to see whether or not you can take your family with you – only to discover that you can't. Should you take the job?

This scenario may seem unlikely, but it's happened to me enough times to realise that there's a mechanism at work here. It's almost as if the Universe, God, or a deity of your preference, picks up your Wish List and says, 'So this is what you really want, is it? So you wouldn't be the slightest bit interested in …' and ka-zaam! The total opposite of what you want is laid out before you, for the taking.

In moments like this I treat it for what it is.

A choice.

This is an opportunity to examine your heart. To think carefully about whether or not the items on your Wish List are things that you *really* want, or things that you *should* want. In short, it's time to be honest with yourself.

Whether you take the job in Dubai (or whatever your equivalent would be) is, of course, entirely up to you. And in my experience, decisions like this usually require a great deal of soul searching, usually when there's very little time to do anything of the sort. Worse still, even once you've made the choice there's nothing to stop the Universe (God, etc.) coming back and asking you again, and again, and again, each time raising the stakes. That just seems to be how it works. So it's important to keep in mind the original question:

What is it that you actually want?

How Is Any of This Nonsense Supposed to Improve My Life?!!?

Ok, enough talk about 'the Universe'. Let's roll up our prayer mats, exchange our orange robes for civilian clothing, and think seriously about getting a haircut and having a shave. Some people just aren't in touch with their inner hippy.

Those same people will struggle with the whole concept of Wish Lists. And though I've done my best to show you that there are some very real, proven psychological mechanisms at play that underpin what some describe as 'the law of attraction', it still feels like hocus pocus to many.

These people don't want to leave anything to shadowy parts of their psyche. Pointing their life in the right direction isn't enough. They want a step-by-step guide telling them how to get from A to B – how to get what they want. They need control, dammit!

And I can understand that. Because I'm one of them. And if you are too, then grab that Wish List, turn the page, and let's talk about how to go about changing your life.

Making Life What You Want

You Can Change Your Life

Does this sound familiar?

6am. The alarm goes off.

Surely it can't be 6am already? Surely not!

You reach for your watch. It too says it's 6am. Amazing. What were the chances? Both your alarm clock and your watch are running several hours fast.

Your partner nudges you in the ribs.

'It's six o'clock.' It is? It really is? And that's not good news because you know from experience that your partner is never, ever wrong.

An hour or so later you're sitting in your car. The radio burbles in the background, but you're listening to the rhythmic sound of the windscreen wipers whilst you stare at the brake lights of the car in front. After a while those lights go out and the car moves forward a couple of feet. You move your foot from the brake, squeeze the accelerator, take up the slack, and then stop again.

It's at this point that a thought floats through your mind. A thought that you will have several more times before you get to work, and numerous times throughout the day. It's a thought that you have so often you barely even notice it any more: 'There must be more to life than this.'

Here's something that you might find hard to believe:

YOU CAN CHANGE YOUR LIFE.

One caveat: 'You can change your life' isn't quite the same as 'You can have the life you want.' I'm not saying you *can't* have the life you want – I'm just saying that it might take several 'changes', perhaps even many, *many* changes, to finally get to where you want to be. But so long as you have 'choices', you can make 'changes', and if you can 'make changes' you can move your life in the direction you ultimately want to go. And whilst the last section was all about the 'figuring out what you want your life to be like', this section of the book is all about the 'moving'.

Turning Wishes into Goals

Grab your Wish List from the last section. In fact, don't even bother with the whole list – the only thing we're interested in (for now) are those top three wishes.

What we're going to do in this section is to take those wishes, and turn them into *goals*.

A lot of my friends dislike the idea of setting themselves personal goals, like it somehow takes the private part of their life, the part that is supposed to be about relaxing and having fun, and turns it into 'work'. Which, as we all know from General Unhappiness Reason Number One, is the mortal enemy of fun and relaxation. There will be those of you who are already resisting this part of the book. You'll be telling yourselves that you've 'tried setting goals before'. That 'it didn't work', or it 'could never work', or that you're simply 'too busy'.

If this is you, then you have my sympathy. I too used to sit in traffic on the M25, morning after morning, listening to those self-help Tony Robbins CDs and wondering whether I'd enjoy them more if I wound down the window and tossed them, Frisbee-like, over the edge of the bridge and into the River Thames far below me.

If you're considering doing a similar thing with this book let me strike some sort of bargain with you. Stick with me for a few more pages. Chances are you will have never set goals in quite this way before – *even if* you've listened to Tony Robbins or countless other gurus. And even if you have, 'setting goals' is only the first step. Crucial, yes, but only in the sense that getting into your car and knowing where you want to go is the crucial first step to any car journey. Later in this section I'll introduce you to a slew of tricks and tools that'll help you turn those goals into reality and prevent them from being nothing more than a pointless list of 'nice to haves', but first we need to talk about 'wording'.

The Vital Importance of 'Wording'

So you have your top three wishes. Surely to make them goals we just declare them as such and hey presto! Job done!

Not so fast, Buster.

To be goals, real goals, we need to infuse them with power. We need to give them the ability to inspire you, move you, prod you, poke you, *irritate you* – whatever it takes, in fact, until they're no longer goals, but Statements of Fact: descriptions of how your life has become.

And how do we achieve this magic?

With words.

Let me introduce you to my friend Anne. She's an odd person. She actually liked the idea of setting goals! There wasn't any arm twisting involved. No sooner was she introduced to the concept than she came up with this list:

1. Be nicer to the kids
2. Listen to more live music
3. Lose weight

These are, on the face of it, very worthy goals. Worthy. But not particularly *useful*. Let's make them better.

Step 1: Getting Personal

Right now Anne's goals are a little anonymous. They read
like slogans. And whilst creating posters that read BE NICE
TO YOUR KIDS might work, it's a little extreme. Let's save
the World War II style advertising campaign for when we're
desperate. Instead, we can boost the effectiveness of the goals
just by adding two simple words – 'I will'.

1. I will be nicer to the kids
2. I will listen to more live music
3. I will lose weight

Now when we read these goals out loud they're no longer
meaningless slogans, or commands, they're *commitments*. By
saying them, even in your head, you're making a promise.

Don't take my word for it. Try it out. What's the one
thing in your life that you would really like to change but you
know in your heart you probably never will? Quit smoking?
Walk the dog each evening? Phone your mother once a week?
Now, plug the words 'I will' in front of whatever it is you've
just thought of and say it out loud.

Do it now.

Ok, ok, you don't *have* to say it out loud – just say it in
your head, but put this book down for a second and do it.

Done it? Ok. But did you *notice how uncomfortable it makes you feel?* Did you notice that little knot in the pit of your stomach, or the niggle at the back of your mind, or the voice in your head that's saying 'Yeah right'? That's the kick back. That's the part of you that's *resisting* the change. That's the little kid in you who used to lie on the floor screaming when you didn't get your own way. All we've done is add two words and suddenly there's a part of your psyche that wants you to quit right now! Believe it or not, that's progress!

I have a friend who says, 'Behind every no entry sign there's a door.' By placing those two words in front of your goals you've created a door.

Step 2: Being in the Moment

If you think your psyche had a problem with 'I will', just wait
and see what kind of fuss it'll make if you replace 'I will'
with '*I am*'.

When we do this to Anne's goals they look like this:

1. I am nicer to the kids
2. I am listening to more live music
3. I am losing weight

Perhaps the first thing to notice here is that you can't just
swap 'I will' for 'I am'; other words have to change too, and
that's because we're changing whole sentences from ones
that talk about this dim and distant point in the future when
we'll be nice to kids, where we're surrounded by live music,
and our excess weight is a thing of the past, to sentences that
describe things that have happened or are happening now.

Suddenly our goal about being nice to the kids isn't an
aspiration any longer – it's a reality. It's happening in the here
and now. We're no longer dreaming about how our days will
be spent listening to live music, it's something that happens
regularly. And we're no longer looking forward to shedding
those pounds, we're … hang on a second. I still don't like that
last goal. 'I am losing weight'? We can do better than that.

3. I have lost weight

Much better. Nobody wants to be losing weight. Losing weight is a drag – we want that weight gone!

'But,' Anne might say to me, 'it isn't true.'

'What's not true?' I would reply.

'The sentence – it doesn't make sense.'

'How so?'

'I haven't lost weight! I'm not nice to the children! And I'm not listening to live music!!' And then she'd probably shake me by the shoulders and I'd be forced to slap her to calm her down.[22]

Of course it's not true. Yet.

What we're doing here is borrowing a principle from hypnosis which says that the subconscious is a highly suggestible portion of your psyche. If you're told something often enough, and with enough sincerity, you will eventually believe it. This in turn will have a knock-on effect on your behaviour, and the choices you make.

You may have heard this referred to as 'brainwashing', which sounds a lot more sinister than it really is. In reality we do this to ourselves all the time.

Can you really brainwash yourself? Yes, you can. By setting our goals in the present, as if they're already fact, we're programming our subconscious to align our reality with what we want.

---

22 Relax – I wouldn't slap her. But I might be forced to stuff a cream cake in her mouth.

Resistance Is Futile

Still struggling with this? Who's still feeling some pangs of resistance? Let's talk about that.

Another peculiar function of the large, walnut-like sponge in your head is the job of maintaining the status quo and keeping you exactly where you are. It's a defence mechanism. A kind of inbuilt 'If it ain't broke, why fix it?' process. Everybody, to a lesser or greater degree, has an in-built resistance to change.

My personal resistance to change is incredible. Just wearing something a little different will have that voice in my head screaming at me, telling me that I'm totally bonkers, that no good can ever come of this radical change of image. I've learned to recognise this voice. I use it to determine whether or not an idea or a course of action might achieve something. If I feel the resistance I know that the idea is likely to lead to change in my life. If I feel nothing, then it'll probably have no effect at all. Perverse though it might seem, it's become part of my mental tool box for making decisions.

So perhaps the true reason for your resistance to writing goals in this way, whether you've realised it or not, is because you *might actually get what you want*, and part of your psyche doesn't want that to happen.

Feeling the resistance?

Excellent.

Let's move on.

Step 3: Making Them Measurable

So let's take another look at those newly worded goals of my friend Anne:

1. I am nicer to the kids
2. I am listening to more live music
3. I have lost weight

Having reworded them you might think that we've significantly increased the odds of Anne achieving them, but you'd be wrong. Whilst the new goals might be enough to motivate my friend into a frenzy of kid pleasing, music listening and weight losing activity, *how will she know when a goal has been met?*

For instance, let's take the last goal – 'I have lost weight'. If this were my goal, could I meet this goal by simply skipping dinner tonight? Tomorrow morning I would doubtless be a few grams lighter! Goal achieved? 'Of course not,' I hear you say. 'That's cheating.' Is it?

Let's take goal number two: 'I am listening to more live music.' If this were *my* goal and I went to one more concert this month than last month, would that be enough to meet this goal? Given that last month I didn't listen to any live music, surely I've only got to see one band and I'm home and dry.

Then again, two months ago I went away to Glastonbury (the music festival) and saw more than a dozen bands. I had such a great time it's the reason I set this goal in the first place – so given this, how many bands do I have to see, and how frequently, for this goal to be achieved?

I'm lying, of course. It's not my goal – it's Anne's. I never went to Glastonbury, and the idea of sleeping in a tent, in a cold muddy field, live music or not, is not my idea of a good time. That's why I'm creating the following goal:

> PETER'S NEW PRIMARY GOAL:
>
> I HAVE NOT BEEN CAMPING,
>
> AT ALL,
>
> IN THE LAST YEAR
>
> (31ST DECEMBER, THIS YEAR)

I am reasonably confident that I'll achieve this, because I know exactly what it is I have to achieve (zero camping) and by when (end of this year). Does Anne know what she has to achieve, and by when? No.

Hang on, you might say – if Anne set the goal 'I am listening to more live music' then she'd have a fair chance of knowing when the goal was achieved. Maybe all she really wants is to be able to recall the last time she saw some live music – and for it to be recent enough that not only can she remember what she wore, but she still owns the outfit.

Likewise with the weight loss goal – surely on the day that she finds her clothes are so baggy that they weigh more than she does, she can declare this goal met. So why complicate things?

But notice what we've done here. Without even meaning to, we've worked out what our success criteria are for those two goals – Anne's clothes won't fit any more, but they will be the same clothes she wore to see a band not so long

ago. That success criterion should be written into the goal –
without it we can never be sure if the goal is met.

To illustrate the point further let's have a look at Anne's first
goal – 'I am being nicer to the kids.'

Goals like this are extremely difficult to quantify. How
will Anne know if she's being nicer to the kids? Having
come from a business background my initial reaction would
be to look for some sort of data source. When it comes to
live music and weight loss there's a set of scales in Anne's
bathroom and her social calendar hangs on the kitchen wall,
but I don't think she keeps a record of the times she's lost
her temper with the kids. So unless she's the sort of person
who writes that stuff in a journal ('Dear diary, once again I
completely lost my rag after little Johnny fed the goldfish to
the cat') the only thing she's got to go on is *memory*.

What's your memory like? Personally I have a hard time
remembering my name. Pinned to the wall by the front door
is a list of things to check before I leave the house. Seriously.
That's not a joke. My wife made it for me after the hundredth
time that I came back to the house to collect my phone, or my
wallet, or my iPod. And those were the times when I could
actually get back in because I'd remembered my keys. But I
digress. The point is, can anyone really remember every spat
they've had with the kids? Really? What, every one?

This is why working out the success criteria for your
goals, *as you set them*, is essential. It forces you to face issues
like this long before they become issues. And in the case of
this goal there are really only two ways to ensure that Anne
can measure it when the time comes:

1. She keeps a log of all the times she loses her temper
    with the kids, or
2. She writes a better goal!!

I don't recommend keeping a list of arguments. In a book
that's all about becoming happier, counting the number of
arguments you have with your kids (or spouse, or boss, or
anyone) is, once again, focusing on what you *don't want* – the
arguments, the spats, your short temper – as opposed to what
you *do want* which is ... what exactly? *What is it you want?*
More quality time? More fun? More laughs? Is that a 'yes' I
hear? Then let's chuck out Anne's horrible negative goal. I've
seen Anne with her kids and she's a great mum! That nasty
goal made her sound like some wicked old crone and that's
simply not true. All she wants is more quality time with her
children – and who could blame her? – in which case, the
goal should look more like this:

1. The kids and I are doing something fun, every week
(31st December, this year).

Now that's a goal I can get behind! It's positive, it's
personal, it's written in the present tense, it's definitely
measurable, and it has a deadline.
Deadlines. Let's talk about that.

Step 4: Setting a Deadline

So Anne's revamped goals now stand as follows:

1. The kids and I are doing something fun, every week
(31st December, this year)
2. I see some live music at least once a month
(31st December, this year)
3. I fit comfortably into my old jeans
(31st December, this year)

You'll notice that they have a deadline assigned to them. Why is that?

A goal without a deadline really isn't anything more than a 'milestone' – something that you plan to pass someday. If a goal is open-ended then it's something that you can put off till tomorrow, or the next day, or maybe next week. And putting goals off defeats the object. You might as well start each one with the phrase 'Won't it be nice when …?' Whereas if a goal has a deadline then it becomes something you can *fail*.

Contrary to what you may have heard, failure – or more accurately, the fear of failure – isn't necessarily a 'bad thing'. No one likes failing. Failure makes you feel bad. And generally speaking people, even people who wouldn't describe themselves as competitive, will do anything they can to avoid that feeling. Most of the time fear is the very thing that gets us to do something. It raises our heart rate, our pupils dilate and it gets our body ready to 'fight' or 'take flight'.

It makes us do something.

Take my track record, for example. I used to set five goals at the start of each year – three primary, and two in reserve (call me optimistic!).

At the end of 2008 I managed to achieve two.

At the end of 2009 I achieved one. Maybe one and a half.

In 2010 I achieved … none.

On the face of it this looks like dismal failure. However, three years later *all five* of those 2008 goals had been achieved. So, although I failed to meet the lofty heights I set for myself in the time scales I initially wanted, I did achieve my 2008 goals *eventually.*

You might think that this adds strength to the argument that some goals could be 'open-ended'. Especially if the goal itself isn't, strictly speaking, time dependent. Why put yourself under unnecessary pressure? Because the pressure *is* necessary – the deadline introduces the possibility of failure, and the fear of failure is what drives you to take action.

Have you ever seen the UK TV show *Grand Designs*? Each week slightly smug but nonetheless likeable presenter Kevin McCloud follows a couple as they attempt to build their dream house.

'And when do you expect to be moving in?' asks Kevin at the start of each show. To which most couples usually say 'Christmas' or 'Summer' or 'This time next year' or some other date that seems as though it was plucked from thin air. If memory serves me correctly, there's only been one couple who have ever managed to meet their deadline – most have nothing more than a shell of a building when the self-imposed moving-in date appears.

However, every now and then Kev meets a couple who waft away his question and tell him that *there is no deadline*, that *it'll happen when it happens*. They usually smile at this point, mentally patting themselves on the back for avoiding the trap of self-imposed pressure and heartache. Forty-five minutes later in TV viewing time, and eighteen months or more in real time, they still haven't got anything that even vaguely resembles a house. Instead they're knee deep in mud, living in a leaky caravan, and sharing a port-a-loo with a dozen slow-moving builders. They're certainly not smiling. And Kevin's smugness has reached new limits.

Setting a goal such as 'I have built my dream house' isn't a goal until it has a deadline. Without a deadline you're never in any danger of failing the goal. 'I have built my dream house *by the end of the year*' – now that's a goal I can respect, because even if, come December, you only have the foundations built and a big pile of bricks in the corner, at least you have the foundations and a big pile of bricks!

Your goal's deadline is the day you're going to either pat yourself on the back, or give yourself a stern talking-to.

It is the day of reckoning.

So to make sure this day doesn't come and go unnoticed you should put it in your diary.

You do have a diary, don't you?

What's wrong?

Feeling some resistance?

Step 5: Penalties!

Occasionally the 'fear' of failing a goal isn't enough.

My deadline day comes around – and what do ya know, I haven't made my first million, I don't own a yacht in the South of France, and I'm still waiting for Kylie to call. I failed my goals. Big bloomin' deal.

This tends to happen when there really isn't a consequence if the goal isn't met. Life without Kylie or a yacht or a million quid might be a little less exciting than I'd like, but it isn't *unbearable*. The trick therefore is to introduce a penalty.

It took me about six years to write the first draft of my novel. Despite the fact that I dreamt of being an author, and that part of this merely required the ability to sit down and put one word after another, it took an extraordinary amount of effort to motivate myself into doing so. It wasn't that I didn't know what to write, or that I didn't like what I was writing, it was that there was always *tomorrow*.

Even after I made finishing the first draft of my novel a goal (written in the present tense, with a deadline), I still failed dismally. The facts were that the consequence of not writing the novel just didn't hurt enough.

Then one day I decided that I would donate £100 to charity each month I failed to complete a chapter. I couldn't afford £100 a month. Did it work?

No.

A month went by. I wrote nothing and, as a consequence, I donated £100 to charity. It hurt. But it didn't hurt enough.

Then my accountant queried the £100 payment. I told her what I was doing and, being a woman who knows a lot about the movement of money, she told me that the experience of 'doing something good' was offsetting the pain of losing the money. To alleviate this problem she would not only decide who the charity would be, but she would keep that information confidential, and future 'penalty payments' would be made payable to her. She also declared that as she was my accountant I had very little choice in the matter. It was a case of 'Do this, or find another accountant.'

Another month went by. I wrote nothing. Again.

Then, to my horror, I was duly summoned by my accountant and told I would be taking her to lunch (which I had to pay for) and to bring any completed chapters – or my cheque book. When no chapters were forthcoming I had to write out a cheque for £100. No explanation for my failure was required – indeed, my accountant was quite sympathetic, and I got the distinct impression that she would be quite sympathetic on a monthly basis.

To this day I don't know what charity (if any) the money went to. But I do know this: it was the only time it happened. The first draft of my novel[23] was completed within six months.

---

23   *The Good Guy's Guide to Getting The Girl.* Despite the title, it is, I assure you, a work of fiction.

Step 6: Rewards!

Remember we talked about how people fall into two distinct groups? Those that 'run away' from things, and those that 'run towards' things?

A 'running away from' approach to life is great for avoiding sabre-toothed tigers. It's also useful when it comes to creating penalties for your goals. Dream up something you really don't want[24] – make that your penalty. Job done.

Every now and then I come across someone from the *other* group. Someone who naturally 'runs towards things'.

There aren't many of these people around. Presumably most were eaten by sabre-toothed tigers many years ago. They're also unlikely to be reading this book given that, in my experience, they're optimistic, have a sunny disposition, and can be quite successful. These people tend to harness the power of focus without even trying, which, if I wasn't such a charitable person, I would find distinctly annoying.

They don't, however, respond to penalties at all well. It just doesn't have the same motivating effect, and in some cases it can be crippling. These folks need 'carrots' rather than 'sticks', because sometimes goals, no matter how worthy they may be, just aren't carroty enough.

---

24 Reader Lynn suggests volunteering your time: gardening for a family member, hand washing your boss's car, etc.

If you're such a person – if you get excited about the idea of earning a 'gold star' at the end of a task – then go ahead and use the 'penalty' logic in reverse. Dream up a series of treats or rewards and assign them to your goals. Heck, why not do both?

STOP! ACTION POINT!

Re-write your three goals

Rewrite your three goals as follows:
- Positive statements (so that the mind focuses on what you want, not what you don't want)
- Personal statements ('I am' at the beginning)
- Written in the present tense (it's happening now or has happened)
- Make them measurable (how will you know when the goals have been met?)
- Give your goals a deadline (a realistic deadline – but not one in the far distant future)
- Make a 'day of reckoning' appointment with yourself – put the deadline in your diary
- Attach a penalty if you need one
- And maybe a reward

Making Your Goals 'Happen'

Annoyingly, no matter how well written they may be, goals don't achieve themselves.

The first year I set myself goals (2007) I failed spectacularly to achieve any of them and for one stupid reason: having set them, I never gave them another thought.

I set five goals on January 1st, and didn't look at them again until January *of the following year*. It took me an entire twelve months to learn the bloomin' obvious: I had to put some effort in!

This is basically the same problem with any list you might make – be that a Now List, a to-do list, or your goals. Unless there's a corresponding process in place to make you look at that list and do something with it, the list will remain a list.

Fortunately for you, when it comes to goals, there are plenty of 'processes'. Let's start with a biggy ...

Goals Day

Hello? Goals Day? Could this be the slightly more serious cousin of Boxing Day and Now List Day? Well yes. Yes it is.

Your Goals Day is an entire day you set aside, once a month, or every other month – maybe once a week or a fortnight if you can manage it – to work on achieving your goals. This relatively small amount of concentrated effort will make all the difference between achieving and failing your goals.

Now there will be those amongst you who will be gnawing at the corner of this book in frustration (I wouldn't recommend that if you're using an electronic device to read it).

'Another day out of my busy schedule?' you might be saying. 'Are you serious?!'

Yes. Yes I am. And whereas I can sort of understand why you'd resist the concept of 'making time to enjoy yourself', working on your three goals shouldn't be a hard sell.

Those three goals reflect the three things you want most in life. If they don't, then you haven't got the right goals! But assuming you've identified three things that will rock your world (or at the very least make it a darn sight more enjoyable), anything that gets in the way of your goals should be, by its very nature, less important.

Yes, most of us have to work, most of us have responsibilities, but twelve days out of a possible 341[25] is still

---

25 Twelve days have already been taken by Boxing Day, and another twelve by Now List Day.

a slither over 3.5%. You spend ten times that amount of time asleep! You probably spend more than twelve days per year just sitting on the toilet! Now that's a sobering thought.

If you seriously can't commit a whole day once a month, then commit half a day, or one day every other month. Or maybe an hour each day. Whatever works for you. And if you are in this situation then I seriously recommend creating a goal to regain control of your life! (Suggested goal: 'I am able to dedicate one day a month to working on my goals (31st Dec, this year).')

But before we fall out over your insanely busy schedule let me sell you some of the benefits. Whilst Goals Day isn't necessarily 'fun' (it feels more like work), it does nonetheless give you a fantastic sense that you're taking control of your life and doing something about it. A day spent on goals is hugely empowering. It's rare that I don't finish a Goals Day feeling like my life has been nudged forward just that little bit more, sometimes a lot more. For that feeling alone it's worth the investment.

Rules of Goals Day

There are, of course, some rules:

Firstly, your Goals Day should be a regular occurrence. I used to only manage to have a Goals Day once a month – I'd have preferred once a fortnight. But if I'd had a Goals Day less than once a month I'd have got seriously jittery.

By 'regular' I also mean 'planned'. Once again you should make an appointment with yourself. In your computerised diary/calendar (now, you do have a diary … don't you?), create a new appointment and set it to repeat every X days/month.

Secondly, what happens when Goals Day coincides with your significant other's birthday? What then? Cancel Goals Day? No no no no no! As with Boxing Days and Now List Days you can reschedule a Goals Day, but you can't cancel it. If this means that by the end of the year you have 12 Goals Days all stacked up next to each other, well that's unfortunate, but so be it.

Let's have a quick recap on what Goals Day is supposed to be about.

This is a day set aside for doing whatever you can to nudge one or two of your goals further.

You might like to split the day into two – work one goal in the morning, and a different goal in the afternoon. This isn't a hard and fast rule, and it might be something that you want to play by ear, but working on one goal all day long can be draining to say the least.

For some people that's pretty much all they need to know to kick off a blur of frantic list making. Those people will start building 'Gantt charts', they'll know what the 'milestones' are, and what should and shouldn't be on the 'critical path', and they'll have already decided who's going to be blamed when the 'deliverables' fail to be ... well ... delivered. The rest of you won't have a clue what I'm talking about.

I could write a huge section on how to break each of your goals down into smaller chunks, and how to work out what those chunks might be – but someone far more skilled than me has already done it.

If you can, get hold of a copy of *Getting Things Done* by David Allen.

Getting Things Done is a practical, easy to follow, no-nonsense guide for creating a structure in your life to *move things forward*. If someone decided to sit down and write the 'handbook for human productivity' this would be it.

It's had a hugely positive influence on my life, albeit in a very simple, no-nonsense way. It's one of those books that I keep having to buy over and over again because the friends I lend it to *never* give it back. That's how good it is! And I wish I'd written it first.

Right now on Amazon.co.uk I can see that there are at least a dozen (second-hand paperback) copies on sale for less than a fiver – trust me, it's well worth that and the delivery charge you'll pay.

However, whilst you're waiting for the postman to bring you your copy, let me lift one tiny piece of advice from Mr Allen's excellent book and share it with you now.

Determining Your Next Action

Whether you want to climb Mount Everest, be the president of the United States, or create a time machine, there are always a finite number of steps between 'here' and 'there' – you simply need to figure out what they are.

Quite often it's not even necessary to know all the steps before you take them – you merely need to know what the *next* step should be.

For instance, want to do something nice with the kids each week? Maybe your next action is to book that time into your diary or start a list of things you and the kids can do. Want to listen to more live music? Maybe your next action is Google local music venues and get a copy of their forthcoming events. Want to lose that spare tyre round your waist? Maybe the next action is to get a copy of *How To Eat Loads and Stay Slim*[26] by the fabulously slender Della Galton and … me!

Let's have a crack at this now.

Take a quick look at your goals and ask yourself this question: for each of the goals you want to work on, what would be 'the next step'?

If several answers come to mind, jot them all down on a piece of paper, then set about doing the one that seems the most logical. If that leads you nowhere, go back to your list and try the next idea.

---

26 Find out more at www.howtoeatloadsandstayslim.com

Some typical 'next actions' are:

- Find out how much something costs, or get quotes
- Find a place that does the thing you want
- Break your goal into smaller steps
- Get a book on the subject
- Google!

If you're *still* struggling to think of your next action, then I humbly suggest that what you might need to do is find someone who can tell you.

For instance, my good friend Karen recently decided that she was going to set about realising her long-term dream of opening a Therapy Life Centre. She set herself a goal. Booked in some Goal Days … and promptly got stuck.

'What,' she thought, 'do I do next?'

Her solution was to invite some fellow therapists round for a brainstorming session. By the end of that afternoon she had a pretty clear idea of what she had to do to make the centre a reality.

There are very few things in this world that haven't been done before. With a little effort it's nearly always possible to find someone who's either done what you want to do, or would have some ideas on how to go about it.

Ready to start achieving those goals and changing your life? Let's do it.

STOP! ACTION POINT!

Book regular Goals Days into your diary

Remember:
- You can move Goals Day – but you can't cancel it
- On your Goals Day:
  - you may like to work one goal in the morning, and a different goal in the afternoon
  - ask yourself what your next action is, then set about doing that action

Goal Minutes

Whilst Goals Days are extremely powerful, they're not the complete answer. They're maybe 57% of the answer. And whilst your goals are probably very different to my goals, personally it would be utterly impossible to achieve just one of my goals with only twelve days' effort a year, regardless of how concerted that effort was. It takes more than that. Much more.

Fortunately, though, I don't necessarily need more time in the form of *days*. Sometimes I just need an extra five minutes, but an extra five minutes at *just the right moment*. Sometimes I need those five minutes when I'm at a party and find myself talking to someone who, if I just remember to ask them the right questions, could be the very person I've been looking for to help me build that new website. Or maybe I need those five minutes when I'm walking past the local adult education centre when for weeks I've been meaning to phone up and ask someone to send me an evening class prospectus. Opportunities like this occur more often than you think – you just have to be able to spot them when they happen.

Remember how we talked earlier about 'focus' and how the brain works? How, when you've decided what car you're going to buy, you suddenly start seeing that same car everywhere? These next couple of steps are designed to tap into that part of your brain and keep your mind focused on your goals, so that when those crucial five minutes appear, you spot them and spring into action.

Got a Wallet?

Most people own a wallet, or purse, or some other item to carry around their payment cards, dog-eared receipts or, if you're really retro, cash.

If your wallet is like mine then it might have a small see-through pocket where you're supposed to put a photo of a loved one. Ditch it. Not the loved one, just the photo.

On a small piece of card or paper, just big enough to fit that space, write down all your goals or, if they won't fit onto such a tiny piece of card (they probably won't), the one that's most important to you, and place it in your wallet. What we're trying to do here is create something that will remind you of your goal each and every time you look in your wallet.

(If you can't bring yourself to ditch the photo, then see if you can engineer it so that the photo and your goal reminder share the space)

This is a very simple idea but one that really works.

You might be tempted to think, 'I don't need to do this – there's no way I can forget what my number one goal is.' But you're missing the point. This idea, and the ones that follow, aren't some sort of 'aide memoire' – it's much more subtle than that. What we're creating is your own personal *subliminal advertising campaign*. We're going to bombard your subconscious with images and reminders so that the 'focus' mechanism in your head is permanently on the lookout for anything that applies to your goals.

So imagine you're standing at the bar, paying for a drink. As you reach for your money your eyes register the small piece of card with your number one goal written on it.

'My polo shirt business has doubled its turnover. 31st Dec, this year.' You take out a twenty-pound note and hand it to the barman, at which point you notice that his polo shirt has the name of the pub chain embroidered on the breast. I wonder where they get their polo shirts from, you think to yourself.

'Here ya go, mate,' says the barman as he hands you your change.

'Thanks,' you say. 'By the way – have you got a telephone number for your head office?'

Got a 'Primary Location'?

Most of us spend our days in just one or two locations. Whether that's a desk, the inside of a delivery van, your spot next to the conveyer belt, or your kitchen and home, a significant portion of your day is probably spent in just one place. Wherever that may be, you can take the general principle of the 'card in the wallet' idea and make a bigger, more elaborate version to suit the space you work in.

What you come up with will, of course, depend on you and your primary location. So if you spend most of your days at home you might like to take a large sheet of coloured paper, write your goals on it in big colourful letters, and stick it to the fridge. If you have young kids – and especially if your goals are shared by the whole family – you could get them to help you decorate it. (My niece never needs much encouragement to get up to her elbows in glue and glitter!) On the other hand, if your kids are older (or you can't be bothered with all that mess), buy some magnetic letters and spell out your goal on the fridge door.

If you're very creative and practical, you might like to
make something you can put in a picture frame; something
that you can put on a desk or hang somewhere prominent.

If you're less hands-on, but own a computer, you
could use it to find a picture on the internet (maybe via a
Google image search) that sums up (one of) your goals,
then use whatever software you have (maybe Photoshop, or
PowerPoint) to add your goal's text on top of it. For example:

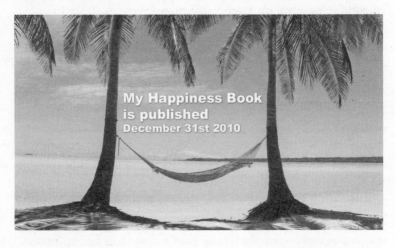

Once you've done this there are *numerous* web-based
services that, for a few pence (really, pence!), will turn your
image into a poster (for your college bedroom), a key ring
(to hang in the van, or put your keys on), a mouse mat (for
your work desk), postcards (to put inside your locker), even
a handbag! Wherever you work there really isn't an excuse
for not having some kind of imagery to remind you of your
goal(s), frequently, throughout the day.

Whilst you're sitting at your computer, what's your computer background (the wallpaper) of choice? A sunset? A picture of your dog? Why not use that image you just created? In fact, why not make an image for each of your goals and then use something like 'webshots' (a very cool, totally free piece of software available from webshots.com) to change it daily?

I even use Windows Scheduled Task manager to open my three wallpaper images so that they are the first thing I see when I switch on my computer monitor.

Obviously, if you work alongside other people and your goals are very personal, or you're just a very private person, these ideas might not appeal to you. There are two things I'd say about that. Firstly, to preserve your privacy try creating something that will remind you of your goal, but without using any words – just imagery. So long as you know what the image represents, the effect on your subconscious will be the same. Secondly, so what if your colleagues know! If they're nice colleagues I encourage you to let them in on your goals. Trust me, nothing motivates you more than knowing you've got to give a progress report every time someone sees that image on your desk.

Either way, do this right and pretty soon you won't be able to go through your day without your computer, fridge, locker or wall gently reminding your subconscious what to focus on.

But we haven't finished yet. Your eyes aren't the only way to absorb information.

Got Ears?

A while back I suggested getting into the habit of reciting your top three wishes (which have now been re-written as goals, making them all the more powerful) as you walk up the stairs, blow-dry your hair, drive to work, or something else you have to do every day.

Now there will be those amongst you, my fellow self-help book junkies, who will recognise that what I'm really talking about here are 'affirmations'.

Affirmations (sometimes portrayed in movies as a guy standing in front of a mirror repeating phrases like 'I am successful, *I am successful*') cause many people to raise an eyebrow – people either love them or hate them. I used to be firmly in the latter group.

However, remember how I mentioned that your subconscious is very suggestible? That if it's told something frequently enough, it will eventually believe it? Which in turn will have a knock-on effect on your behaviour and the choices you make? Interestingly, this includes all the times you tell yourself that *you're stupid, you don't feel well,* or *you don't like something*. There's been a surprising amount of research on the subject of 'self-talk' and it turns out that negative internal chatter is far more damaging than you might think.

Recently a big dirty ginger cat moved into my neighbourhood. It's a nasty-looking brute. It's the kind of cat that scowls and looks as if it should be wearing an eye patch. But worse than that, it's taken a particular dislike to my petite moggie.

For several weeks now I've had a water pistol at the back door ready for the moments when I hear my cat hurtle through her cat flap with Evil Ginger Cat in hot pursuit. The last time this happened was about two o'clock this morning. I was woken by the now familiar sounds of two cats either side of a plastic flap, batting it back and forth with their claws and paws whilst they hiss and howl at each other. I grabbed my robe, ran down the stairs, grabbed my water pistol and, as I opened the back door, fired off two shots into the darkness.

When I poked my head outside I could just see the shadowy image of the ginger cat, silhouetted at the end of the garden, just out of firing range. But I was ready for him. I reached into the bucket by the back door and grabbed one of the water-filled balloons that I'd prepared for this very moment, and I lobbed it with all my might in his general direction.

As I did so, I felt my ring – my wedding ring – slide off my finger, and a second or so later I heard it tinkle on the paving slabs, somewhere in the garden. In the darkness.

This morning, when the sun eventually came up, I went into the garden and spent a good half hour looking for the darn thing. A small silver coloured ring, against small grey slabs, covered with a layer of dead leaves, in the rain and the bitter cold. Not surprisingly, my hopes of ever finding my one and only sentimental piece of jewellery weren't high, and as I worked my way from one end of the garden to the other and back again, I muttered the words, 'I'm never going to find this thing,' under my breath.

Now this is God's honest truth, but eventually I realised what I was doing – telling my mind that I would not find the ring! So I changed the words. 'I *am* going to find my ring.' I said it once. Then again. And again – and as I carried on looking, within about five seconds (I managed to say the phrase about five times) I found it! I was so surprised I actually spent a few seconds checking the engraving inside the ring just in case I'd found a completely different platinum wedding ring amongst the leaves in my garden.

Coincidence? Maybe. I'd go as far to say probably. But I've come across similar examples time and time again.

Like the friend of mine who has a blog no one can remember the name of, because it includes the word 'forget' in the web address.

Like the actor I worked with recently who throughout rehearsals failed to exit when he was supposed to, because his cue line (which was intended to be ironic) was 'I'm staying right here.'

Or like my friend Della, who took weeks to finish a short story because she'd entitled it 'You never finish anything.'

They're all examples of times where words that people say, or read, get lodged in the subconscious, and influence their behaviour. Powerful stuff.

This being the case, negative self-talk is a *really* bad habit to get into. And given that there's often a bunch of people lining up to point out our faults, why be one of them?

Instead, I encourage you to become your own fan club and use self-talk (affirmations) to your advantage. When you say your goals to yourself, say them out loud. Say them several times. Say them like you mean it.

You may find it easier to remember what to say (and the fact that you have to say them at all), if you have them pinned to the mirror, or the dashboard, or the bottom of the stairs. Personally, I read them out loud when I switch on my computer screen each morning.

More powerful still is to *record* your affirmations, then play them back to yourself each day, and repeat what you hear. This prevents you from rushing through your daily affirmations. If you're musical, put them to music, but if you're like the rest of us, just read them slowly and clearly into a tape recorder.

If you own an iPod or other MP3 player, and have the ability on your computer to record your voice, you could go the whole hog and create yourself an 'audio screensaver' – a thirty-second audio snippet that pops up now and again and reminds you of your goals. It's a little like having a motivational commercial break whilst you're listening to your fave tunes.

Here's how:

1) Record yourself reading the goals and create an MP3 file. Keep it short: thirty seconds or so. I usually read through my five goals twice.

2) Import into your iTunes[27] music library.

3) Set up your MP3 player (I use the 'playlist' functionality in iTunes) so that your 'self-talk' file appears periodically. I have a 'driving' playlist that I use in the car that always includes my self-talk file.

4) Create a rule with yourself that you will not skip this file when it plays if you're the only one who can hear it.

5) When the file plays, if you're alone, repeat the goals out loud to yourself.

---

27 Or equivalent.

Now there are those of you out there who will have decided that I've just gone too far and I'm clearly bonkers. You're not alone. My brother was stunned into silence when I told him about this, which, if you know my brother, you'll know is a rare thing indeed. But believe me, it works. Whether you use 'impromptu iPod affirmation sessions' or you merely recite your goals every morning, by using self-talk you're giving your psyche something positive to work with.[28]

---

28 An excellent book on the subject of affirmations and self-talk is *What to Say When You Talk to Your Self* by Shad Helmstetter.

STOP! ACTION POINT!

Use the power of focus by creating a subliminal advertising campaign for your subconscious

Try any or all of these ideas:
- Put a reminder of your goals or primary goal in the photo part of your wallet or purse
- Create images applicable to your goals and place them where you will see them during the course of each day
- Use affirmations. Say your five goals out loud to yourself each day. Record them to make the experience more powerful

Finding Yourself a Goals Partner

Right after Goal Days, and filling your life with subliminal (and less than subliminal) reminders of your goals, having a Goals Partner is probably the next most effective way of achieving your goals.

My Goals Partner is Denny. In fact, Denny was the one who got me interested in the concept of goal setting in the first place. If you're not enjoying this part of the book then Denny's to blame. At least in part.

Let me reiterate something – Denny was the one who got me *interested* in goals. She didn't introduce the concept to me. Having read more than my fair share of self-help books I thought I knew all that I needed to know about goal setting – enough to know that it wasn't for me – but Denny was the first one who made it fun.

'I've set myself five goals for next year,' she told me one January night, over a curry.

'You've set yourself goals?' I said

'Yeah,' said Denny, mopping up some curry sauce with a strip of naan bread. I was stunned.

'Why?' I asked.

'Because I'm fed up with my life the way it is.'

'Setting yourself goals is a little extreme, though, isn't it?' She shrugged.

'Not really,' she said.

'But what if you don't achieve them?' I asked.

'Then life will stay pretty much as it is, I guess. From that perspective I can't really lose.' I thought about this for a second or two.

'Maybe I should set some goals,' I said.

'Maybe you should,' said Denny. 'What would they be?'

For the rest of the meal we chatted about what each of our goals would be, and why. It was fun. And that made a huge difference – setting my goals with someone else was *fun*. It wasn't some crazy thing I was doing on my own, in a vacuum.

This same technique is used by clinics to help people quit smoking. Once you've made a commitment to yourself in front of someone else, your chances of success increase dramatically.

That said, the first year Denny and I set our goals we didn't actually discuss it again until the following year. And that was a missed opportunity. Especially as we meet for a curry at least once a month. Now we quiz each other on our goals progress each and every time we pay a visit to the curry house. It doesn't necessarily dominate the conversation, but it's as much a part of the curry experience as ordering poppadoms, or the hot towels at the end.

Stop! Action Point!

Consider finding yourself a Goals Partner

Got a friend out there who'd be happy to be your Goals Partner? Give 'em a call. Invite them over for a meal. Lend them this book if you have to.[29] Once you've persuaded them, remember to:
- Meet up regularly to discuss your goals
- Keep it fun

---

29 Lend? What am I saying!? <u>Buy</u> them a copy!

The Day of Reckoning

Breaking Open the Champagne!

So today's the day! The day when your goals expire. Hopefully you've achieved one or two – maybe, just maybe, all three?

Let's consider that for a moment. You've achieved something that was _so important to you_ it was amongst the top three on your original Wish List, and was subsequently made into a goal! Well, big pat on the back for you! Congratulations! You should celebrate. Seriously – you should. It creates positive reinforcement in your psyche. The better the celebration, the more you'll want to achieve future goals.

So, what are you going to replace it with? I'm serious. You're on a roll now, so dig out that Wish List and write yourself a new goal to replace the one you've just crossed off.

And this time, dare to think bigger. Much bigger.

Oh, and feel free to skip the next couple of pages.

What's up? Why are you still here? Why the long face?

Oh.

I see.

Close, but No Cigar ...

So, you failed one of your goals.

Maybe two of them?

All three?

I'm sorry to hear that – though not as sorry as you might think.

So what happens now? Should you declare the whole 'goals' experiment a disaster and have a ritual burning of this book? Definitely not! Not when you could re-sell it on Amazon or give it to charity. No, get rid of this book if you must, but if you give up on goals now you've only done half the work.

Firstly: You Failed, but You're Not a Failure

This is important: whilst you failed to achieve the goal, if you made time to work on your goals, and if you moved yourself forward even one inch, you, the person, are *not* 'a failure'.

'Failures' are people who don't get out of bed in the morning. 'Failures' are people who don't even try. But each and every time you worked on your goals you were achieving something, so let's not start branding ourselves with a big fat F, because as we already know, that kind of negative self-talk is toxic and unhelpful.

Let me reiterate this:

> **YOU FAILED TO ACHIEVE THE GOAL,**
> **BUT YOU ARE NOT A FAILURE.**

Secondly: You're Supposed to Fail (More Times than You Succeed)!

The not so funny thing about setting goals is that some of the time, perhaps even *most of the time*, you *should* fail!

This could just be me, but I'm not particularly motivated by 'easy goals' – goals that I know I have a good chance of achieving. They don't even feel like goals – more like boring items on my to-do list.

I had a friend who, on January 1st, set herself the goal of joining a gym. By the end of the first week she'd achieved it. Was that really a goal? Was that really one of her *top three* items on her Wish List? Shouldn't joining the gym have been part of a much larger goal to improve her health and fitness?

In my mind a goal should stretch you. A goal should be ever-so-slightly out of reach. With most of my goals I know that my chances of success are extremely slim, though the chance is there.

You Don't Have to Succeed First Time!

A lot of people have this inbuilt drive to succeed, *first time*. What a terrifying prospect! There are very few things in life where you're only allowed to have one attempt.

And – whether you're learning to drive, learning to paint, running a marathon, overcoming your fear of approaching women – whilst it hurts to fail, there isn't actually anything physical preventing you from trying again. And again. And again.

It depends on the goal but in general I'm not particularly keen on *succeeding first time*. There's very little to be learned from a first-time success – I'd rather fail but know how close I got, and why.

Which brings us rather nicely onto the next and *most important* point about failure.

Failure is 'Feedback'

You can learn a lot from failing your goals. Sometimes you discover a new way of *not* doing something. Other times you find out you're on the right track, but you need more time.

And if you then take that information and use it to help you make better decisions, thereby increasing your chances of success, was it really failure? This might be a hard thing to comprehend, but that 'failure' can be a very good thing *if* you treat it properly.

The most important aspect of failure is the new information it gives you. So, grab yourself some paper and ask yourself the following questions:

1. Why did I fail? Did I run out of time? Or was there another reason?
2. What have I achieved? Would I have done so without this goal in place?
3. What do I need to achieve this goal? More time? Something else?
4. Is this goal still relevant? Does it need re-writing? Should it be replaced with a different goal?

The answers to these questions serve to do three things:

1. They should console you – by concentrating on what you have achieved
2. They should inform you – by identifying the reasons why you failed
3. They should inspire you – so you know how to set subsequent goals

In many ways the concepts of success and failure are far too rigid, far too black and white, far too binary. Maybe you weren't 100% successful – but were you 80%? 50%? 25%?

'Real failure', so they say, is not 'the falling down'. Real failure is 'not getting up again'.

Now, pick yourself up – and start again.

But the Word 'Failure' – Arrgggghhh!!!

My assistant, Jules, suggested I try to find another word for 'failure'.

'It's such a negative word,' she said. 'It implies you weren't 'good enough'. Can't you tell the readers that there is no failure? They just didn't, well, 'achieve it'? The word 'failure' makes me itch!'

It makes you itch, eh? Now that is interesting. Tell me more about this itch. Is it annoying? Does it make you feel uncomfortable? Does it make you want to wriggle about? Do whatever you can to get rid of it?

No one likes failure. When we fail it causes us pain. I've watched my six-year-old nephew throw objects across a room in frustration when he lost a game of Snakes and Ladders. The experience of failure is so upsetting that many people develop a fear of failure.

Fear, pain and, indeed, itching, are all mechanisms your body uses to motivate you. Surely anything that motivates you is, at least in part, useful?

Resetting Your Goals

What? You thought goals setting was a one-time deal?
Au contraire, my friend, au contraire.

By identifying why you achieved or failed your goals
you're equipped to write smarter, more specific, or maybe
utterly different goals. But the important thing is to cash in on
all that new information and make better ones.

Avoid, if you can, simply resetting an old goal. The
definition of 'insanity', so they say, is trying the same thing
over and over and expecting a different result. You should
have lots of new information to feed into the goal setting
process.

Take, for instance, one of my goals for 2010:

My Happiness Book is published
(Dec 31st 2010)

At the time that I set the goal, I'd hardly started writing
this book, let alone given much thought to how I would
publish it. By the end of 2010 not only did I know what I
needed to do to get this into your hands, but I also had a
pretty good idea of where I wanted to go after that. So my
revised goal for 2011 looked like this:

'HOW TO DO EVERYTHING AND BE HAPPY'

IS AVAILABLE IN THREE FORMATS,

AND SELLING REALLY WELL

(OVER 1,000 COPIES A MONTH, IN TOTAL, ANY FORMAT),

WHILST I BASK IN THE SUCCESS OF THE WORKSHOPS

(AT LEAST ONE A MONTH, EVERY MONTH)

DEC 31ST 2011

Interestingly enough, as I write this now (March 2012) it's worth pointing out that I also failed the revised goal! At the end of 2011 the book was only available in two formats, not three, and I'd only managed to run one measly workshop. I had however sold over 5,000 copies. Not bad.

By the time you read this however, this book will be available in three formats, I'll have sold 10,000 copies and my workshops will be a regular occurrence. Will that be enough to achieve my number one goal for 2012? Oh come on. Have I taught you nothing? Of course it won't!

I like to set my goals at the start of each year, and review them at the end. For me, that works. This might make them sound a little like 'resolutions', but resolutions are something entirely different. 'I will give up smoking' – that's a resolution. 'I have given up smoking (Dec, this year)' – now that's a goal.

You don't have to set them yearly. Maybe quarterly works for you. Maybe it's dependent on your goals. The important thing is not how often you review or renew them, *it's that you do*.

Working with goals – that is, having them in your life – is something that gets easier the longer you do it. You develop a habit. A mindset. After a while you start to look at everything you're doing in relation to how it sits with your goals.

In a very real way, your goals force you to decide what's important to you and move you in that direction. They give you purpose and vision.

It's true what they say:

'WITHOUT VISION THE PEOPLE PERISH.'

STOP! ACTION POINT!

The Day of Reckoning

If you fail a goal
… ask yourself the following:

1. Why did I fail? Did I run out of time? Or was there another reason?
2. What *have* I achieved? Would I have done so without this goal in place?
3. What do I need to achieve this goal? More time? Something else?
4. Is this goal still relevant? Does it need re-writing? Should it be replaced with a different goal?

If you achieve a goal
… congratulations!

1. Go back to your Wish List (or create a new one).
2. Set yourself a new goal.
3. This time, think bigger.

Use all this information to set new goals.

Potential Goal Problems

Ok, settle down, settle down – from experience I already know that there are probably 50% of you out there who are sitting, arms folded tightly across your chest, scowling at me. Of all the concepts discussed in this book goal setting is the one that people wrestle with most. So, allow me to try and address as many of those common goal-related problems as possible.

Words and Terminology
'Goals', 'wishes', 'failure' – some people have a real problem with these words.

'Goals' sounds too corporate, too managerial, too board-room, too annoying, too schoolteacher-ish …

'Wishes' sounds too flaky, too holy, too hippy, too girly …

And let's not get started on 'failure'! We already know how that brings some people out in hives!

If you're struggling with these, or any other words, then *change them.* Pick something else. You have my permission to go through your copy of the book and change the word 'goal' to 'target' – or 'wishes' to 'wants', whatever works for you. The important thing is not *the word*, but the concept behind it. If you can't hear 'failure' without wanting to scratch, then *change it* – how about 'Personal Target Re-assessment Opportunity'?!

This goes for any of the lists, days or concepts elsewhere in the book. Don't like 'Boxing Day'? Can't stand 'Now Lists'? Re-name them.

If you think of any good word alternatives feel free to send them to me and I'll list them on the website for other word-challenged readers – but please, don't let a word stop you from getting the most out of goal setting or this book.

Too American

It's important to realise that I am British. True – I don't live in a castle, I don't have a butler, I don't particularly like battered fish wrapped in newspaper, I'm not a huge fan of roast beef, I can't stand football, I certainly don't refer to it as 'soccer' – but other than that, most of the stereotypes are probably accurate.

I have worked for numerous American companies over the past fifteen years and some of their culture may have rubbed off on me – some. But I've *never* skipped my lunch, worked late into the night, high-fived my colleagues, or winked at them whilst saying, 'Good job!'

That said, our 'cousins' across the pond are, as a nation, just a whole lot better at 'self-improvement' than we Brits. And for decades American authors have taken ideas that work, re-branded them, and presented them to the book-buying public as groundbreaking and new. So if you've ever read, watched or heard anything on 'goal setting' or 'the Law of Attraction' it's possible that the ideas presented in this book are going to feel – well, 'American'.

So here's a suggestion: join me. Join my little crusade to reclaim these sensible, practical, powerful ideas and re-present them, without the fluff, without the mystique, and with a distinctly European flavour.

I Just Don't Have the Time for Goals or Goal Days!
Hang on – didn't I address this way back at the start of the book? And then again under Now Lists? And yet some of you are still convinced that to apply everything you've learned in this book you've somehow got to conjure up 36 days out of thin air.

Let me be clear on this point:

YOU DO NOT NEED TO

FIND 36 DAYS

TO MAKE THIS BOOK WORK!

What's needed here is a little 'time accountancy'. Take all the important things you're *currently* doing and shuffle them around to fit in one of the three days mentioned in this book.

So let's recap what each of the days are and how they fit into your oh-so-busy life.

Boxing Days – Boxing Day can usually be 'reclaimed' from activities, particularly weekend activities. Some people get up on Saturday and go shopping, or wash the car, or watch football on the TV, and for no other reason than it's Saturday! If that's you, one Saturday a month can now become Boxing Day. And if you wake up on that Boxing Day and you *want* to go shopping, wash the car, or watch the match, then go right ahead.

Now List Days – These don't have to be whole days. Not if you're planning. You can break them down and have Now List evenings, lunchtimes, even breakfasts. And if you're not *planning* – if you're actually ready to do an item on your list – that might be a perfect vacation activity rather than spending another day sitting around the pool.[30]

Goal Days – Goal Days are twelve measly days out of 365 to be spent on the three things that you want most of all in life.

Let me say that again:

The three things you want <u>MOST OF ALL</u>!

Before you bought this book one of two things was happening. Either you were completely ignoring all the things that are now on your Wish List, in which case you were probably deeply unhappy, or, more likely, you *were* struggling to address those three things, albeit in your own way.

Long before I discovered the power of goals I spent many an evening and weekend struggling to turn my writing, and other interests, into something that might bring in a few quid. If you've been doing the same, then all that time you currently spend working on your dreams and ambitions can now be *reallocated* as Goal Days (or evenings, weekends etc). Maybe it's not 12 *days* a year – maybe it isn't that structured – but it's time that you don't have to 'find'. All you need to do is start using it properly.

I understand that you're busy. I do. And I appreciate that if you work for someone else, and/or you're a parent, you probably can't juggle your diary quite as effectively as I

---

30 If 'sitting around the pool' is really important to you, add it to your Now List or Wish List.

can. I get that. But whilst I've never been a parent, I wasn't always self-employed. And whilst life is hardly fair at the best of times, one thing that does seem to be consistent is that anything worth having in this world usually comes at a price. And it's usually a lot more expensive than you initially thought. Happiness is one of those things. To get it you have to work. Hard!

Before I bust your chops any further, here's a suggestion that my friend Wendy came up with.

If you find yourself struggling to juggle your time, perhaps this is a good opportunity to look at what's currently eating up your minutes.

In Wendy's case, a considerable amount of her day was spent working through what appeared to be an ever growing pile of ironing, until one day she made the momentous decision that, as there were things in life more important than ironing, ironing was no longer going to be a daily activity. Furthermore, if her three teenage children and partner disagreed, then they were welcome to assist whenever they wanted.

Too Rigid!
One of the problems with writing a book like this – one that's based heavily upon personal experience – is that all the ideas and suggestions will work perfectly, if you happen to be me.

Of course, you're not me. So when it comes to goal setting (or indeed anything else in this book), for goodness sake use your head. If setting _yearly_ goals doesn't work for

you, set them at other times! One of my friends sets them as
and when her life dictates.

If three goals is too many, try two. Or one. If you have
enough bandwidth to cope with more than three, try four,
or five.

And though I've said it already I'll say it again – if I
come across like a schoolteacher, then I sincerely apologise.
I'm just passionate about this stuff. And the more I see it
working for people, the more passionate I become.

Oi! I Thought You Were Going to Address the Difference between My Wish List and My Now List?

Ah yes. Thanks for reminding me. Let's recap.

You remember we were questioning the difference
between your Now List and your Wish List and whether
it's ok if something makes both lists – well, now that we've
talked about goals let's think about this again.

The short answer is no, it doesn't matter. If you want to put
something on both lists and that makes sense to you, go right
ahead. What goes on which list is far less important than
understanding how each list works and why.

Imagine you head up a corporation with two groups of
people at your disposal. Over there, in the factory building,
you have your Now List Department, whereas over here, on
the fourteenth floor of your corporate headquarters, you have
the Wish List & Goal Division.

The Now List folks will diligently work through anything
and everything you give them, albeit at their own methodical

pace, trying to get as many things done before – well, before the whistle blows and they rush home to their families.

The Wish & Goals operatives, on the other hand, will *consider* any request you throw at them, but until it's passed rigorous internal scrutiny to see whether it should be adopted as one of your corporation's three goals, won't do very much with it. When it *is* a goal however, they'll assign a deadline, introduce rewards and penalties, create a poster campaign, organise affirmation sessions, work overtime, and generally throw every resource they have at it.

So then, let's take that wish you had earlier to climb Mount Kilimanjaro. Which group of your people do you want to give that to?

Final 'Wish List and Goal' Thoughts

Whilst you have choices (and there are *always* choices, if you look hard enough) you can make changes.

Maybe not everything, and maybe not overnight, but given enough time and consistent effort you can move the mountain of your life from where it stands now to where you want it to be or, at the very least, a good deal closer.

It was Benjamin Disraeli, British Prime Minister, who said, 'Success is entirely dependent upon constancy of purpose.' He was so right.

Figure out what you want, set yourself goals, and begin.

You can change your life.

Putting It All Together

The End Is Nigh

Guess what! You've almost finished the book!

Yes, I know – you were hoping that this was an index or the acknowledgements section, or something else you could skip.

Well, if your life has become a blur of Boxing Days, Now Lists, Wish Lists and goal-related activity – congratulations! – you probably don't need to read this section. My work here is done.

If, however, you need a little more help and a few pointers on where you should go from here – this section is for you.

Grab a pen and lots of paper.

For real this time!

What Do You Want?

Start thinking about what you really want, in all areas of your life. And use that information to make the following lists:

Your Potential Boxing Day List

Your Potential Boxing Day List contains things that you *could*, if you felt so inclined, do on a Boxing Day. You need to be able to update it as and when an idea occurs to you, so put it on your phone, in the back of your Filofax, or anywhere it's likely to be close to hand. Don't wait until you have an idea before you start this list – the very act of creating a blank list will start your brain thinking of things to put on it. This list should not contain items that need pre-planning – put those on your Now List. On the other hand, if there are items on your Now List that require no pre-planning whatsoever, move them to here!

Your Now List

Your Now List contains all the things you'd like to experience 'before you die'. Like your Potential Boxing Day List it's a work in progress; you're going to add things as you think of them and cross them off when they've been done. And again, don't wait until you have an idea – start a blank list now.

Your Wish List

Your Wish List contains all the things you want in your life, or want your life to be. Think about every aspect – work, personal, spiritual, physical – everything. Think big. Think small. If you have wishes that are reliant on or related to each

other, write those down too. There's no limit on the number of
wishes you can have – they merely have to comply with the
laws of physics. Go crazy. Write down absolutely everything.

Your Goals List
Your Goals List is very short. It consists only of your top
three, most important wishes, but re-written in the form of
goals. Goals should be:
- Positive statements (focuses on what you want, not
  what you don't want)
- Personal (starting with the words 'I am …')
- Written in the present tense (it's happening now or has
  happened)
- Measurable (so you know when the goal has been
  met)
- With a deadline (a realistic deadline – but not one in
  the far distant future)
- … and finishing with a penalty, and/or a reward

Focus and Evidence

Having started your lists, reinforce the ideas by feeding your subconscious.

Collect Inspirational Pictures

Spend some time (though not too much) trawling the internet, or flicking through magazines, for any images that inspire you or remind you of your goals, or things you want.

Mementoes and Souvenirs

Out having fun with friends? Keep a paper napkin, pick up a card when you pay the bill, and hold onto that ticket stub. Having the best vacation ever? Send *yourself* a postcard! Pick up a pebble from the beach. Collect anything that can act as evidence of all the times you've enjoyed yourself.

Tools of Your Trade

There are a variety of objects that you might need to help organise all this list-making and collecting activity. They are:

- A couple of cork boards – for inspirational imagery, and your 'trophy board'
- A printer's tray, an empty glass jar, a shoe box – for items you can't pin to the board
- Image software – to make wallpapers and screensavers
- Sound software – to record affirmation MP3s
- A diary

You do own a diary, don't you?

Making It All Happen!

You didn't think I'd finish this book without another diary mention, did you? And there was me thinking we've got to know each other so well.

Grab your diary and put the following appointments in it:

Boxing Day

Maybe once a month – whatever works for you – perhaps the 26th of each month (there's a wacky idea).

Don't worry too much about diary clashes for the moment, you'll sort those out later. Right now it's more important that Boxing Day is in your diary on a regular basis.

Now List Day

Or Now List half day, or lunchtime, or breakfast, or whatever works for you, as regularly as you deem it necessary.

Remember, this is the day when you'll either be doing something on your Now List, or doing things towards making those things happen.

Again, don't worry too much about diary clashes at the moment.

Goals Days

Have Goals Days once a month – or twice if you can. Goals Days are the most important out of the three, and are the ones that'll ultimately make the biggest impact in your life.

Arranging Your Diary

Right then – Boxing Day is now in your diary, as well as Now List Day and your Goals Days. Now it's time to enter everything else – birthdays, anniversaries, appointments, personal holidays, public holidays, reminders, *everything*. Anything that can use up your valuable time should be in that diary.

Flick back to the 'How To Use Your Diary' section early on in this book (or visit the website) for an exhaustive list of time-devouring events.

If you've done this right there's a good chance you're staring at the most chaotic diary you have ever seen. There are probably clashes and overlapping appointments everywhere! Don't panic. Take a deep breath. Crack those knuckles and get ready to play god with your life.

Starting with 'today' and moving as far forward as you feel the need (a couple of weeks usually works for me), move the appointments around until you've eliminated all the clashes. Don't start cancelling things – that defeats the point of the exercise. But if there's a Boxing Day right on top of your optician's appointment, *move* Boxing Day to a spare slot. If you have working days taking place at the weekend, find an appointment you'd rather do at the weekend and *swap* them.

After a little practice you'll find that you get quite good at this. And it goes without saying that all of this is a LOT easier if you can see a whole week at a time and your diary is electronic.

The diary shuffling exercise isn't a one-off task, it's an ongoing process. This isn't a sign that things aren't working – quite the reverse. This is how the process should work.

You might also discover that it's rare to be able to add a new appointment without creating a clash. Again, this isn't a problem. This shows that your time is *valuable* and that you need to decide what it's spent on, rather than giving it away.

Living by Your Diary

Now that your diary is planned, start living by it day to day.
Get into the habit of checking, each morning, or the night
before, what you have planned for the next 24 hours. This'll
take some getting used to – particularly if you're the sort of
person who currently gets out of bed, or arrives at work, and
basically does whatever comes to hand.

Remember, you can still make last-minute changes to
your schedule – so if you discover it's not possible to do
whatever the diary has planned for you, *swap* (don't cancel)
today's appointment with a different one.

Now that you're letting the diary dictate how you manage
your time you may notice that it's not as easy to say 'yes'
when someone asks if you can make a meeting or if you can
spare some time to help them out. Again, that's evidence that
the diary is working. Agree to help or meet that person if you
want to, but only if you can fit them into your busy schedule.

One final diary tip. Nobody else has to know what's in your
diary. In my experience showing people your diary is never
a good idea. It merely opens a discussion about what you've
chosen to spend your time on, and you'll probably find that
people who want a piece of you rarely feel as passionately
about your need for a Boxing Day as you do. Keep your
diary – or portions of it – private.

Advanced Diary Tips – Other 'Days'

Having introduced this concept of pre-arranged 'days', you
might want to experiment with creating days of your own.
This is particularly powerful if you work for yourself, but I've
known colleagues who do the same with their working day at
Mega Corp Ltd. Here are some days that sometimes feature in
my diary (remember, these are only examples – they may not
work for you):

Default Day
Default Days are days specifically set aside for my 'default'
activities, which are:
- clearing the post and in-tray,
- then my email inbox,
- before returning to the master to-do list.

I used to have a default day once a week. Now I've
broken it into two default 'evenings'. Like all my 'days',
default days/evenings can be moved, but never cancelled.

Also, on the rare occasions that I wake up and find that
there's a blank space in my diary I treat it as an extra default
day.

Writing Day
A Writing Day is the day when I do whatever writing or
editing needs to be done. That probably sounds obvious, but
because writing is something that I need to 'get into' (it's
difficult to dip in and out of writing), it's also one of those
tasks which I tend to put off. I have a tendency to look at the

next item on my to-do list and say to myself, 'I'll just do X, Y and Z first.' Hence Writing Day.

Maybe your equivalent would be a Cleaning Day, or an Admin Day, or Personal Finances Day.

Promo Day
A large part of what I do actually involves promoting my writing and other activities. Promotion is one of those activities which don't seem to reap any immediate dividends – so whilst none of my promo tasks is particularly onerous, it's extremely easy to leave it till tomorrow as 'one day is unlikely to make a huge difference'.

Unfortunately tomorrow – as the song says – never actually arrives, so the promo work never gets done. For this reason I invented Promo Day.

I soon found that an entire day of promotional activities was too much to cope with, so Promo Day is now a half day, several times a month.

Recovery Day
Recovery Days are inserted as and when I think I'll need them. For instance, if I know I'm going to be flying home from a trip, or having a particularly boozy late night, the following day might be allocated as a Recovery Day.

This might seem extraordinarily decadent. How luxurious that I can afford to take an entire day to recover from a social event! However, too many Writing Days, Promo Days, Goal Days etc. were effectively being lost through trying to operate with a head full of porridge. It seems far more sensible to accept the fact that I need to recharge.

Things still happen on Recovery Day. It's just given over to doing all the mundane tasks that require very little brain power or physical exertion.

Friends and Family

To ensure that Peter doesn't become all work and no play I started to reserve days for friends and family. Note that I don't necessarily know in advance which friend or family member I'm seeing on the days allocated – but these appointments exist in the diary to prevent the time from being swallowed by something else.

When a friend or family member suggests we meet up I find the next *friends and family* day and shuffle my diary accordingly.

'Random Acts of Kindness' Day

One of my newer ideas that I've been experimenting with is a day dedicated to Random Acts of Kindness. Now before anyone starts nominating me for a Nobel Peace Prize or anything like that, let me assure you that my motives are purely selfish.

I recently came across some research by happiness researcher Sonja Lyubomirsky. She's discovered that there's scientific basis to what your mother always told you was true; it's better to give than receive.

In one study, people who were asked to spend one day a week doing five small random acts of kindness for others ended up significantly happier than those in another group who were doing one act a day.[31]

It's certainly food for thought, and was enough to make me want to trial the idea in my own diary-obsessed way.

Having invented these 'days' I pre-book them into my diary – just as I do Boxing Days, Now List Days, and Goals Days. I go through this process once a quarter because whilst a particular 'day' might work for me now, in a few weeks' time it might not, or I might need more of them.

As you can imagine, my diary looks pretty crowded (see example on the following page), but it gives me a level of control over my life that I previously never had. I no longer wonder where the time goes, because I'm the one deciding what I spend my time on – in advance.

One word of warning – if you decide to run your diary like this be sure to build in some slack – days when there's nothing planned at all. Otherwise it's almost impossible to move things around, and there will always be unexpected appointments that need to be slotted in.

---

31 For more on this and many other intriguing social studies take a look at the excellent book *59 Seconds* by Professor Richard Wiseman.

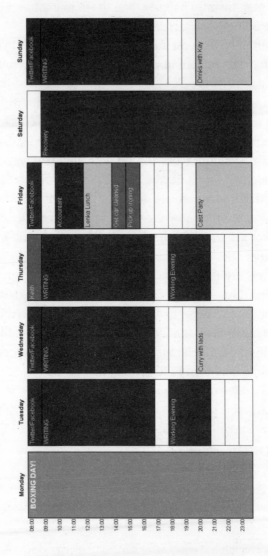

Exhibit C: A page from my 'scary' diary

A Day in the Life of You

So … you've made lists, and you've organised your time. I thought it might be quite helpful to finish up with examples of how three of your 'Days' might look, using my life as an example.

Boxing Day
The following is an entry from my Boxing Day journal. (Yes, I keep a Boxing Day journal![32] So sue me!) This particular Boxing Day followed the last night's performance of _The Importance of Being Earnest_ (which, if you've been paying close attention, you'll remember was on my Now List):

- Got up a little later than usual. Boxing Day initially cancelled because a friend needed to be picked up from the airport so I swapped it for a Now List day. By 9:40am I'd made treacle tart (which was on the Now List). Felt good.
- My friend cancelled the airport pickup (!!) so elected to have Boxing Day after all.
- Checked emails and spent some time on Facebook downloading the cast photos.
- Resized partitions to make more space on my 'music' drive.
- I ate two slices of treacle tart whilst watching the movie _The Importance of Being Earnest_ – this was a

---

32   Just to be clear, I'm not suggesting for one moment that you should keep a Boxing Day journal of your own. I only started it recently as part of an ongoing self-experiment – you know what I'm like.

great idea. Thoroughly enjoyed the film knowing all I now know about the play. Tart was a little stodgy.

- After the movie called Mum to discuss the tart.
- Did a little writing – didn't really mean to, just started reading the chapters by my bed, then making notes, then before I knew it I'd ticked off three items on my writing to-do list.
- Had a walk to the shops. Bought stuff to make pizza.
- Sorted through all my old LPs and singles, making a list of the ones I haven't got on my iPod. Then I went and downloaded them all from the Amazon MP3 store and sent a text to Ellen to tell her I had three boxes of records she could have for her vinyl collection. She was chuffed to bits.
- Long relaxing bath.
- Made pizza – from scratch! Base included!
- Decided to watch another movie. Pizza was amazing. Movie was total trash.
- By 9:30pm I was utterly exhausted. Went to bed and listened to audio book.
- Early night.

Now List Day

My Now List Days are only ever a full day if I'm doing something off the list. Otherwise they're half days. This is how one typical Now List (Half) Day panned out:

Now List Item: Go to a 'Pop-up' Restaurant

- Researched restaurants on the internet.
- Signed up to a couple of mailing lists.

Now List Item: Games Evening
- Couldn't get a consensus from my friends as to when would be a good time to host a games evening. Everyone is so busy between now and Christmas.
- Decided to move this to the 'Time sensitive' portion of the list and to try again in the New Year.

Now List Item: See Bill Bailey
- Visited the Bill Bailey site. Again.
- Discovered Bill Bailey is finally back in the UK and performing at the Wyndham in the West End.
- Booked two tickets.

Now List Item: See Imogen Heap at the Albert Hall
- Only a month to go before Imogen Heap is at the Albert Hall.
- Emailed friends to see who would like to go with me.

And that was it! Half day over. You might think I didn't really achieve very much, but from my perspective I nudged four items from my Now List forward.[33]

Goals Day
I split my Goals Day into two and work one goal in the morning, and another goal in the afternoon. I decide on the day itself which of my three goals I work on, depending on which two I want most at that given moment.

---

33 And by the way, both Bill and Imogen were fabulous. The pop-up restaurant was a hoot!

Today is a Goals Day.

This morning was spent working on the website that accompanies this book, whilst this afternoon has been spent finishing this very section!

And am I going to achieve my goal of having this book on bookshelves, and in audio, by August 1st?

No.

Not a chance.

There are only a few more days before month-end, and before this book is anywhere near ready there's a mountain of editing and proofreading and recording and marketing to do.

But I will get there. You know I will.

After all, you're reading it now, aren't you?

You Still Here?

And there was me, thinking that last page would drive you from your armchair in a frenzy of goal setting. Ah, but I can see from the smile on your face that you have no intention of doing so, that today is a day for doing whatever you feel like. Tell me, is it Boxing Day?

And whilst we're on the subject, how's your Now List coming along? When was the last time you created a memory?

I found a website today of a company that does excursions along the River Thames – I'm finally going to see my house from the estuary! And a few weeks ago I got to spend some time feeding lemurs. Again.

Final Remarks

If you learn nothing else from this book, remember this – you have only a finite number of days on this earth, and they may be less than you think. A lot less. Why would you want to spend one moment longer than you have to being less than happy?

The American President John F. Kennedy allegedly told this tale about the great French Marshal Lyautey, who once asked his gardener to plant a tree; the gardener objected, saying that the tree was 'slow growing' and would not reach maturity for 100 years. The Marshal replied, 'In that case, my dear man, there is no time to lose; plant it this afternoon!'

Boxing Days, Now Lists, Wishes and Goals. They're very different trees. But oh, what fruit. Go on – plant yourself a forest.

Best wishes, Peter

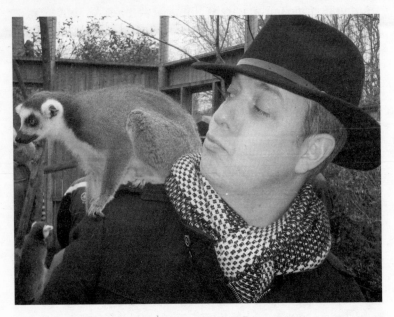

If You've Enjoyed This Book …

I've been ever so slightly overwhelmed with the positive feedback I've had for this book. I mean – I know the ideas work, at least they do for me, but I really wasn't expecting people to get as enthusiastic as they have!

So, this being the case, if you've enjoyed what you read and you'd like to 'spread the word', then here are a few ways you can do just that.

Like the Facebook Page
For starters if you're on Facebook pop along to the Facebook page, www.facebook.com/howtodoeverythingandbehappy, and click the LIKE button (up there at the top).

Your 'friends' will be able to see that you're a fan, and you'll see comments from other readers in your feed, as well as a daily post from myself. Nothing too intrusive, I promise.

Feel free to post a comment or two yourself, or share a photo of you reading your book.

Follow Me on Twitter
If you're more of a twitterer I tweet under the handle @doitallbehappy. The odd re-tweet would be most appreciated.

You can follow me here: twitter.com/doitallbehappy.

Review the Book
Positive reviews are always welcome, and you can leave one on any retailer website from which this book is available.

Got a Blog or a Podcast?

A mention of the book, or a link to the website (howtodoeverythingandbehappy.com) is always appreciated.

If you'd like me to write a guest post for your blog or interview me for your podcast, just drop me a line.

Tell a Friend

And finally, one of the hardest things for any author to achieve is 'word of mouth' recommendations. Next time you find yourself sitting next to someone who's telling you how awful their life is, do yourself (and me) a favour – tell them about this book!

If you can do any of these things, I'd like to offer you my heartfelt thanks. It quite takes my breath away when I think about just how supportive people have been.

And whilst I'm in the 'thanking' mood …

Acknowledgements

Well, this is exciting! The acknowledgements section! It's a little like standing on the podium at an awards ceremony … only without an award, or the applause, or the dinner jackets. Ok, so it's nothing like an awards ceremony. It's more like standing on a street corner shouting at anyone who happens to be walking past – and that's a shame, because there's a small, select group of people without whom I could never have got this book 'out there', and they really deserve the 'awards ceremony' style of acknowledgement. So if you could just imagine the lights, the cameras, the glasses of champagne – I'd very much appreciate it.

In no particular order I'd really like to thank:

My totally fabulous and long-suffering assistant, Jules – for making the really important stuff in my life 'happen', listening to my endless babble and nonsense, reading my 'stuff' (several times, even when it was total rubbish), and generally putting up with me. Find out more about what Jules gets up to when she's not keeping me in line at balloonbaboon.co.uk

Wendy – my dear, dear friend, fellow author, and 'wise and sexy guru' – for her endless passion, and encouragement. For reminding me that there's more to life than we can see with our eyes or hear with our ears, whilst at the same time keeping my feet on the ground. But most of all for keeping me on track, focused, and believing in me when I wasn't so sure. Find out more about Wendy at wendysteele.com

The lovely Della Galton – for putting up with my occasional rants and tantrums, and for being generally wonderful. I could not have got this far without her wise advice and guidance. Find out more about Della, her books, courses and short stories at dellagalton.co.uk

My completely brilliant agent, Becky Bagnell – for her unstoppable energy and enthusiasm, and for believing in me and this book. You can find her at lindsayliteraryagency.co.uk

Becky Glass, Natalie Jerome, and all at HarperCollins. May this be the start of a long and fruitful relationship.

The awesome Alison the Proof Fairy, Author Kerris Stainton and my Marketing and Social Media Guru, Sue Mellor – thanks, ladies.

Anne and Denny – for being hugely influential in the 'Goals' section of this book.

My original 'first readers', Lucy, Lucy, Patrick and Karen – and my second edition first readers, Lynn and Della – for their invaluable comments, thoughts, feedback, support and encouragement.

All the folks who took the time to blog, tweet, 'like' and review this book. This version wouldn't exist without you.

And to you, the reader. For taking a chance on this book and reading all the way to this point! You fabulous, crazy person, you.

Thank you all.

About the Author

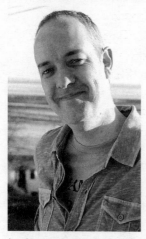

Peter Jones started professional life as a particularly rubbish Graphic Designer, followed by a stint as a mediocre Petrol Pump Attendant. After that he got embroiled in the murky world of credit cards until a freak accident with a zip zap machine (remember those?) restructured his DNA at the molecular level and gave him entrepreneurial powers.

Now, Peter spends his days – most of them anyway – writing. He is the author of two and a half fabulously popular self-help books on the subjects of happiness, dieting and online dating. If you're overweight, lonely, or unhappy – he's your guy.

Peter lives just a few miles outside London with his cat. From his window he can see France and the Eiffel Tower. Or is that Canvey Island Oil Refinery? Hmmmm.

He doesn't own a large department store and probably isn't the same guy you've seen on TV in *Dragons' Den*.

You can find out more about Peter Jones,
his books, speaking engagements & workshops,
at www.peterjonesauthor.com

Praise for *How to Do Everything and Be Happy*

What a great book

A very accessible, practical guide to getting the most out of your life. It covers lots of ideas that I will be trying out over the next few months. However, the book offers these ideas without being in any way preachy or condescending, remembering that people are all different – and offering advice on how you can adapt the ideas to make them work for you. Highly recommended. I really enjoyed it!

Sarah (Chatham, UK), 17 June 2012

No-nonsense practical and friendly advice

This is a great book. It contains helpful methods to make you live a happier and more fulfilling life. The tone of the book is chatty, as if it is your best friend sitting next to you giving advice. I found the diary part and the setting of goals very useful. I am now implementing the 'now' list and 'wish' list. What truly stands out with this book is that whilst chronological in your development, it also takes time out to advise if something has gone wrong. It doesn't steam-roller on to the end, leaving those behind who maybe haven't achieved a goal or stage of the process. Peter dusts you down in a non-judgemental fashion and then continues his journey with you.

D.K. (UK), 2 July 2012

Very do-able

I love this book – it's down to earth, practical, no-nonsense and, best of all, English. Unlike many American-style self-help books, it doesn't promise miracles, just an eminently sensible way to make order out of chaos and make life enjoyable again, with lots of little (and big) bonuses along the way to _____ own life. Thank you,

S. Capes (

Absolutely love this book

I love this book so much. Like a lot of people, I often felt a bit 'meh' about my life. I wasn't miserable, but I certainly wasn't overwhelmed with joy. I didn't want to emigrate, I didn't want to change careers … I just wanted to feel a bit happier with my lot, really. Before I read the book, I'd started to make a few changes. Not massive leaps, just tweaks here and there. By the time I'd finished it, I'd taken a lot of the author's advice and I'd tweaked a bit more. I can honestly now say that I have never been happier. Yes, I sometimes still feel 'meh', but these are fleeting moments, not general discontent. Thanks ever so much for writing it. I work in a library and intend to recommend your book to everyone. Even if they've only come in to use the photocopier.

    Annie Latter (Essex, UK), 20 July 2012

Good, fun, easy read

Just finished the book! It was a great, easy read and I really enjoyed it. It was absolutely perfect for me in simply helping me to realize just how disorganized my life was. Two of my friends are on the 'Happy' bandwagon now, too :) Great job on your book, Peter, and many wishes for your future success!

    Heather (Texas, USA), 27 July 2012

*Read more 5-star reader reviews
at amazon.com and amazon.co.uk,
or at howtodoeverythingandbehappy.com*